# NURSING MNEMONICS TRIGGER 2022

The Most Effective Memory Tricks and
Visual Mnemonic Aids for Nurses to Trigger
your Memory and Crush the Nursing School

# Table of Contents

# Chapter 1

## What are mnemonic memory techniques?

Mnemonics are a way to improve your memory and help it to work better. What exactly are mnemonics? Can you use them to improve your memory? What are three great examples of memory mementos?

I will give you three great examples of mnemonics memory techniques. If you have memorized a phrase, you can write it down or type it on a card and remember it later. For example, the first two examples are: Write the first phrase on a card and write the second phrase on a slip of paper. Memorize this phrase. You can practice this until you can say the word without thinking.

A good mnemonist should always use a "keyboard stroke" or a short, crisp sound when writing a phrase. This creates an association in your mind between the item and the sound made by that stroke. If you start typing the word and then remember it, you may realize that you cannot order the phrase because you have a mental association with the idea. This technique, called typing in a word, is what is called a memorial.

Another excellent example of mnemonics memory techniques is an assembly language. Have you ever been in a meeting where you had to say something like, "The secretary is currently waiting for you in the conference room?" If you never said that, how would you know when you needed to say it?

Another excellent example of mnemonic memory techniques is the language of music. It may not be common knowledge, but actually, piano players use a form of memory known as memory stretching. This means that if you memorize an entire sheet of music, rather than focusing on every note, you create new associations, which improves your ability to recall what you've previously memorized. This technique is also helpful in learning how to play an instrument and improving your speaking voice.

Suppose you were to ask a person unfamiliar with the piano an example of mnemonic memory techniques. In that case, they might tell you that it is simply using critical letters to remember words. While this is an excellent explanation, it does not give you enough information about how mnemonics work. The most effective techniques will take you step-by-step through the process, including songs, hand movements, and phrases.

You might even be familiar with some of these memory strategies already, such as flashcards that include words in song form. Or mnemonics cards, which have pictures that can be used to help you remember phrases or words. But if you were to look at this from a different perspective, would these examples help allow you to remember things? In other words, do they provide information about how things work when used in actual life? And do they make you think about things in a more abstract way? This is what mnemonics is all about.

These memory techniques are designed to encourage you to use the pieces of information you have gathered to help you remember. This is not to say that all of your data is relevant or useful. It may be that you need to revise old information or learn new skills. But having a mental map or list of the relevant parts of the activity can make it far easier to recall the main points. Also, these rhymes and mnemonic devices are not intended to replace books and other reading material. Instead, they are a valuable addition to help you improve your memory skills, mainly if you already use several of these techniques.

# Types of mnemonic techniques

Here are eight types of mnemonic techniques you can use:

- Spelling mnemonics
- Feature mnemonics
- Rhyming mnemonics
- Note organization mnemonics
- Alliteration mnemonics
- Song mnemonics
- Organization mnemonics
- Visual mnemonics

# Spelling mnemonics

A great way to remember words is to use a Spelling Mnemonic. These are mnemonics that aid the memorization process. Mnemonics are a type of memory trick that helps with the quick recognition of words. They work in such a way as to assist you in remembering words, whether you are just reading them or are reciting them. Many of us are not fond of mnemonics because they make us think twice before utilizing the word associated with the mnemonic. For example, let's say that you want to know how to drive a car.

The first thing you would do if you want to learn how to drive a car is to get some sort of guidebook and start looking at diagrams on the covers of the different vehicles. You may even look at some pictures of other models of cars. You can do this to memorize the various terms, parts, and designs associated with these vehicles.

After you have already looked at pictures of cars, you would then want to look at the different Spelling Mnemonics. When you look at the mnemonics, it is essential to pay close attention to the exact spelling of each letter. This way, when you write things out, you will spell out the words that you are trying to remember. If you use an example, you will be able to write out the word "apple". This will take a few tries, but you will finally realize that Apple is spelled as "apy" after several attempts.

Another great thing about these mnemonics is that you will learn all of the specific parts of the word that you are trying to memorize. Many different mnemonics help you understand the pronunciation, spelling, and even the various letters and numbers that go along with the word's spelling. It is straightforward to memorize all of the parts of a sentence if you use the correct Spelling Mnemonics that you have been using before. If you are looking for a quick memorization tool, these can help you out.

Learning mnemonics can also help you to write things out. Sometimes when you type up a letter or a phrase, you do not put the proper punctuation marks around the words you are writing out. By learning the Spelling Mnemonics beforehand, you will see how the correct punctuation should be written out. Then you will be able to write out your sentences and even chapters before you have to write them out.

You might be surprised at the things that will come upon a Spelling Mnemonic. Take, for example, the following sentence. Mary was a pretty red-headed girl. In this example, you would expect the words red-headed and red to be in the sentence. However, if you know the mnemonics, then you will be able to write out this sentence quickly without any problems.

You might find yourself having to look up words that you do not know very well. When you learn the Spelling Mnemonics, you will be able to look at the word and immediately know its definition without having to look it up any further. This can help you to learn things much faster and to write things out more effectively. You will also learn to see patterns much more accessible and understand the different meanings specific mnemonics give you.

If you are trying to learn how to spell, then you should consider Spelling Mnemonics. They can help you out tremendously when you are trying to learn new things. Learning new words can sometimes be a challenge, and using mnemonics can help to make it easier for you. Not only will you be learning new words, but you will be gaining a great insight into how the words were derived from their root words.

# Feature mnemonics

Feature mnemonics are mnemonics that are used to recall words or phrases. They can also be used to remember the names of people or things. A feature mimic is a single thing, such as a word, phrase or name. There are many different kinds of mnemonics.

One type is alliteration mnemonics. These are mnemonics that use certain words or phrases to remind you of the alliteration of the word or phrase. This includes words like "the" or "be." Many English learners prefer alliteration mnemonics over other types. They use alliteration mnemonics to help them with their studying and learning English.

Another type of feature mnemonics is called rhymes. Some people find it hard to remember a new colleague named Bob. To place this new colleague's name, you can use the rhymes feature mnemonic memory technique.

Other types of feature mnemonics are called note organization mnemonics and rhyming mnemonics. Note organization mnemonics will help you remember the central ideas or parts of a poem or a story. It allows you to organize your notes so you know where they're located. You may not know the main idea of a poem, but you'll be able to remember the main words by using note organization mnemonics.

Another technique is known as rhymes. It requires musical devices to teach you how to associate particular words or parts of a sentence with their corresponding elements in a song. Some examples are: If you hear the word blue in the piece "cities", you'll know that the last part, the chord, contains the word society. You can learn the techniques by listening to a song and then trying to remember each note. You can try using the feature mnemonics for note organization in the same way.

The last technique is called alliteration mnemonics. You write down the word you want to memorize while repeating it. For example, if you have the sentence "The man loves his dog", you can form it in the following way: The man loves his dog (alliteration mnemonics) He's going to get the dog (alliteration} Then he'll take the dog (rhymes). You see, by applying different kinds of feature mnemonics, you'll be able to remember all sorts of things. In the same way, using alliteration or rhyming mnemonics, you'll be able to memorize all kinds of things.

That's the overview of the eight types of feature mnemonics. Now let's talk about the examples. To help you remember all the things mentioned, here are eight types of feature mnemonic techniques you can use: alliteration, rhyming mnemonics, alliteration/rhymes, phonetic mnemonics, alliteration/syllabic mnemonics, phonetic/pronunciation mnemonics and spatial/ temporal mnemonics. As I explain below, these all have their uses.

Alliteration - this is a feature-mnemonic technique in use since the start of time. It's like using an acronym with a word that you don't know but which you think fits the description of the item it represents. This technique works well when you don't know the exact word or phrase you want to memorize. For example, if you were looking for the name of an acquaintance, you could use " acquaintance" as a feature-mnemonic device. If you know the first letter of each of the words in the acronym, then you can use "A" for all the acronyms, such as "AJ", "AO", "AR", "BH", "BE", and "BJ". This technique can help you remember lots of stuff, but you have to work with it in a step-by-step manner, starting with the simplest things first.

Acronyms are also helpful when you memorize a sentence and cannot think of the exact term or name. You may find that this technique will work for you. For example, if you have to write down your friend's phone number, you just type it into your computer, and a feature mnemonic will come up. This is not only a speedy way of remembering, but it is also a very convenient way to recall. You won't have to go through the trouble of typing in every possible synonym of your friend's phone number.

Phrase alliteration - this is another feature-mnemonics technique used by many people to remember just about anything. For example, if you were to look up the lyrics to a famous song by one of your favorite artists, you may find that you don't quite remember the words, but you do remember the rhythm. So if you type the words "she rode on a golden rose" into a feature-mnemonic, you will very easily remember the song mnemonic, even though you may not reflect the words to this particular song.

Feature mnemonics can help you to remember just about anything. When you type in a particular mnemonic device, it will usually give you the proper name of the thing you want to remember, the location where you should place it, and the best time to use it. So remember that an acronym, or even a simple phrase, can be handy when memorizing something.

# Rhyming mnemonics

Rhyming mnemonics can be used to help students remember concepts that they have learned. Many of the ideas taught in classrooms fall out of step with what is being taught in most classrooms today. Students tend to focus on the wrong information when they are doing their lessons. This leads to poor test scores, less participation from classmates, and teachers complaining that the class does not move forward as quickly as they would like it to. There are many ways to help students remember what they have learned, but rhymes are the easiest ways to do this.

Rhyming mnemonics are an excellent way for children and adults to remember words or concepts they have encountered before but would like to memorize better. Some people memorize the essential dictionary, while others need to do the work themselves to remember what they have learned. If you find yourself in this situation, try using rhymes as a memorization aid. These can help you to remember things by reading them aloud. You can also write them down and then sing or recite them to yourself as a way to remember them.

Another way to help students remember new information is to use rhymes with further details. Consider a time when you received a letter or package with a new address. You may have already written down this address on your planner, or you may not have a way to remember it.

Rhyming mnemonics can help students remember the great lakes because many lakes in the US are located near each other. For example, those near the Canadian border are near the Great Lakes. This helps students to associate the name with what the lake looks like. This is especially useful in North American English, where the great lakes are often misspelled.

Some teachers will assign homework tasks that incorporate rhymes with lots of different entries. This can help a student learn how to memorize entire phrases. For example, if the assignment requires you to say "Acrostic" and "monarch" while simultaneously forming a sentence, it can help students memorize these phrases. However, using the words "Acrostic" and "monarch" in conjunction with the word "adder" should be avoided.

"Acrostic" and "monarch" are two separate words. Combining them in a sentence would not make sense. Instead, they should be used in a list where the first item is "acrostic" and the second is "monarch". This gives students a visual aid to help them remember the correct order. Another plus for using rhymes with a lot of punctuation is that the letters do not change color when placed after they are correctly pronounced, as with using free form sentences that require placement of the color correct in the parenthesis: "This is a great acrostic".

Rhyming mnemonics are a fun way to help students retain new information. Many high school and college students will create a mnemonic strategy for a new subject name. Each time they use the new term for research purposes or when presenting the information to others, they will use this strategy. These strategies can also be used during discussions. Encouraging students to use these mnemonics during meetings helps them remember the new information. Most high school and college students have never heard the term before attending class.

Using rhymes as a teaching tool has been shown to help children in many ways. Most elementary students learn better from mnemonic devices than they do by simply repeating information. Even advanced students benefit from rhymes and can often remember them quite easily. It is an excellent way for teachers to keep their classes both exciting and compelling. Teachers who choose to implement them throughout the course can then encourage their students to use them in their everyday lives.

# Note organization mnemonics

Note organization mnemonics is an effective way to remember information. They are used by people who are interested in teaching or coaching. These techniques are beneficial for those who are making presentations at conferences or during seminars. Note organization mnemonics use the fundamental law of the mind - the brain likes to associate things with words. Here are some examples of using note mnemonics to help promote memory.

o Notecards - note organization mnemonics make use of the fundamental law of the mind - the brain likes to associate things with words. For example, a notepad is used to remind people of what they have written down. Many beginner speakers often use notecards to remind them of the main points of their speeches. Notecards are not only ideal for lessons, as they can be adapted to many other situations such as press conferences and meetings etc. Another advantage of notecards is that it is straightforward to write down important information.

I before e except after c - this type of note organization mnemonic is an easy way for someone to remember information. Depending on memorization, it is usually written on a card and used at the beginning or end of a speech. This one is perfect for athletes because they need to memorize all the time they play.

o Crosses - cross notes are great as well. They promote recall in a way that lists are often forgotten. There are three examples of this category. If you want to upgrade the memory in business writing, use the classic example of a crossed off-page. If you want to remember information about a person, include a picture. And if you're going to remember your phone number, have the digits.

o Lecture notes - these are the most widely used type of notecards. Lecture notes are so successful as a memory device because they are written in large letters. Therefore, if you have to write something down quickly, it will not be difficult to recall it. When using lecture notes, it's also essential to provide an example of a specific situation where the information will be helpful. Use these notecards to remind you to think about essential things and to promote recall.

o Word mnemonic - use word mnemonic as a note organization mnemonic when working on a sentence, for example. For example, if you are working on a sentence like "His brother hit Joe", you could use the word Mnemonic for "brother" or "hit". The "hits" can be any number of things that indicate how many times the sentence has been repeated. To use a similar example, the word mnemonic could be "The brother hit Joe over the head". This example would be great for remembering the exact order of events that occur in the story.

Note organization mnemonics are handy tools that can be used in classrooms and even in everyday life. Use them for writing and remembering anything you come across. They can help students to recall information more effectively and remember things that they have previously forgotten. Even when we are not actively thinking about something, we can still easily remember it using a mnemonic. Learn more today by exploring the different mnemonics

## **Alliteration mnemonics**

Alliteration mnemonics are a powerful way to help you memorize faster. There are several good reasons for this, the main one being that they allow you to remember better. Alliteration is the repetition of certain words. By using a word that has a lot of meaning in it, you can repeat that word over and over in your head. This makes the information in your memory stick better.

The most important thing about an alliteration mnemonic technique is that you must use one that works well with your other skills. For example, if you are trying to memorize the lyrics to a song, you would want to use a good memory trick such as note organization mnemonics. Note organization mnemonics help you take the information you are reading and convert it into a list of notes. You can also build up to more complicated mnemonics if you are good at it.

As an example, say you are trying to learn how to play the guitar. If you are using alliteration mnemonics, you would probably choose songs with a lot of guitar chords. Now say you want to know which chord is the hardest to play. Your note organization mnemonics could be telling you to look at all the guitar chords that can be played, then tell you the name of each one so you can memorize the easier ones.

Other great examples of note organization mnemonics are spelling mnemonics. If you have a book with many difficult words, you can look up some of their definitions online. Then you can use these spelling mnemonics to help yourself memorize the problematic words, so you don't have to struggle while reading.

Another example of using alliteration or rhyme mnemonics is learning how to solve problems. One of the main factors that keep people from learning how to do something is not remembering what they need to do to get to the result. So if you have a list of things that need to be done but are unsure of how to go about it, an excellent way to remember them is to use a rhyming or alliteration mnemonic. You will also not forget the vital information because you will be using your memory to translate the essential information into the correct pronunciation.

One of the best things about Alliteration mnemonics is that you can use them with any text, even if you are trying to learn Spanish! Since you are being asked to memorize a word or set of words, you can choose which ones to use for each part of the sentence and then have a flashcard ready for each piece. With Spanish sentences, you can make use of the audio feature mnemonics or the picture feature mnemonics. The audio feature mnemonics have the words repeated over, and the picture feature will give you an image that will help you remember the word.

When you are looking at Spanish sentences, you might want to look at song mnemonics. They are very effective because you can associate the words with the melody that goes with them. You will remember the vital information about the music because you heard it associated with the song.

When you want to learn Spanish, you will discover it well by using Alliteration mnemonics. There are various types of these mnemonics out there, and you should be able to find one that you like. Some of these are also known as Spanish Analogous mnemonics. This simply means that they are similar to other types of mnemonics. For example, you might learn about the law of attraction in a way that all the people who read about it will eventually understand. Alliteration mnemonics help you learn Spanish in this way.

# Song mnemonics

Song mnemonics are images or pictures that help us remember things. They use drawings and photographs to remind us of events, and often they rely on a story to help reinforce their meaning. While there are many different types of song mnemonics, bird song mnemonics is one type that has stood the test of time. Here's a look at bird song mnemonics.

Organization mnemonics is a type of memorization technique that many people use. When you learn an organization's mnemonic, you essentially associate it with something you already know but need to memorize to use it effectively. For example, when you look at an address book, you have to look at every one of the names to name them. When you use a mnemonic organization technique, you are essentially memorizing an entire organization by association.

Phrase mnemonics is another example of an organizational mnemonic technique. Using this technique, you will create sentences that make sense but without actually using any words. Instead, you will memorize a word or phrase, spell it out, and then mentally associate it with what you already know. For example, if you see a picture you like, you can turn it into a sentence by transforming it into a phrase.

Another excellent example of a mnemonic technique is ocean blue. Ocean blue stands out as a good mnemonic because it is simple. Instead of looking at a picture and memorizing the words, you will look at it and instantly think of ocean blue. Ocean blue has always been a good mnemonic because it stands out in memory.

There are many more types of mnemonics available. One popular choice is birds. Birds are evocative, and because they can be used in a variety of ways to refer to different types of birds, they can be used in conjunction with other types of bird songs to create a song mnemonic that works for you. You might not immediately know what birds are meant to represent, but you will eventually learn them through the associations you build up over time.

Song mnemonics can help you learn to memorize your phone numbers or address. Even professions like medicine or law require memorization. Without a suitable method of developing a new association, you will find it difficult to remember the details of legal documents or telephone numbers. By using organization mnemonics, you will develop a system in which you can quickly memorize information. Through repetition, you will be able to repeat the appropriate elements of an organization or a document.

In addition to using bird song mnemonics to learn your surroundings and how they relate to birds, you can also use them to identify birds that you happen to see flying around your yard. Many people who have a hobby of bird watching have a great hobby because they have developed a real sense of wonder about the different species of birds they see each year. When you want to expand your knowledge of various species to identify them quickly, you can use mnemonics to help you do this.

Learning to recognize bird songs is something that will remain with you for the rest of your life.
Whether you take pleasure in seeing birds or you enjoy studying and listening to the sounds of various bird songs, you will always find yourself looking at the sky or reading a book about bird songs.
The best way to keep yourself interested in this hobby is to start by memorizing a few of the different bird songs that you can hear when you are out in the open without any other birds in the area. This will give you a good base of familiar sounds to use when you get that call from your favorite bird song. Song mnemonics can significantly assist in this process.

# Organization mnemonics

Organization mnemonics are an essential part of any organization. They provide people with a way to remember what they need to do to accomplish their work. An acronym is an excellent example of a mnemonic device. These are words or names that have special meaning to the person who has them memorized. The use of acronyms is a way to remind people of these names.

An example of an organization mnemonic would be "section," "section head," "project," and so on. The repetition of these words helps people remember the exact phrase or words they need for the task at hand. One can create their set of mnemonics. For example, if you were required to research a document, you could use the phrase "researching historical documents."

Another way to use organization mnemonics is to remember larger pieces of information.
Think of the way you might place a telephone number. You might first have to look it up in a directory or the spellings of the phone numbers that you may know.
This kind of Mnemonic can help you to remember larger pieces of information. Like the telephone number, you might also want to create your own sets of mnemonics for large tasks, like completing a survey, building a house, driving across the US, sailing, and so on.

Another example of an organization mnemonic is to remember the names of people. Maybe you work with someone in a team, or you work with someone in an organization. When you come across the terms of these people, you might want to write the name down to remember it. With the Mnemonic in hand, you can begin writing down their names in the order that you first learned them. This can increase recall considerably.

An easy way to remember words is to imagine the meaning behind the spelling. For example, if you are spelling a word out like a word in a French dictionary, you might want to write the comment out phonetically and sound the word out in your mind. This can also increase your ability to spell the word out by replacing each spelling letter with its corresponding letter in a new language such as Spanish or Chinese.

Another connection mnemonic is to remember where something is. Perhaps you found a dog in the street, but you do not know its name. By spelling out the dog's name associated with specific street addresses, you can increase your recall of this item. Like the dog, another connection mnemonic can be made when the spelling mnemonics come into play.

You might want to memorize a date or time, for example. You can make a date out of it by adding the day, month and year to it.
Another connection mnemonic you might consider for memorizing dates is to think about what you will have to do on the day, month and year in question. Remembering the items you need to do during said dates can give you an advantage in time management.

There are many types of mnemonics, which can be used to help people remember things. This variety covers a wide array of methods and products. The trick to remember, though, is finding one that works best for you. Keep in mind that no matter which mnemonic devices you use, your memory never forgets. So, find the one that works best for you and start using it today.

The Fast Scrabble Word Association Test is an effective mnemonic device. It looks like a game, but with a twist. As you choose a word from a grid, you have to fill in the appropriate type of memory device. As you fill in the various terms associated with your choice, you'll have to remember things like the acronym for that particular type of a memory device, the size and shape of that specific type of memory device, and other important information that goes into the formation of the associations.

An example would be: if you were choosing an initial letter of the alphabet, you could imagine the capital letters of all the common initial letters of the alphabet. When you're done with your choice, you simply write the appropriate Mnemonic. For instance, if you wanted to learn the word "cupboard," you would look up "cure" on a web search engine and then type in "cupboard" into the search box.

One example of a commonly used mnemonic would be the initial letters of the first seven coordinating conjunctions. This is useful for learning a large number of phrases in language, for example, "the grass is always greener on the other side." You can also find many free word mnemonics online, including the famous phrase, "the best things in life are free." You can download some of these, such as the initial letters of "freedom," "the power of love," and "work from home." You can print these out at home and take them with you when you go out for the day, so you'll always know where you're going.

# Visual mnemonics

Visual mnemonics are mnemonics that help people remember things. There is a lot of research that shows how our brains remember things. We have more than enough neurons in our brains to keep track of thousands of items at one time. These memories are like short stories that our brains build when we are younger. They are often called "category cells" because they connect certain things like colors, places, and other things that we usually associate with the events that occurred. These mnemonics are great for helping people memorize things.

The most effective Mnemonic is one that does not say anything directly. Instead, it gives some kind of story that makes you think about what you are reading or remembering. For example, if you were learning about the North Pole, you might visualize an ice age so that your brain doesn't have to associate the North Pole with the cold. It might be a good idea to make the visualization as realistic as possible. If your mother had told you about the ice age, it might be a good idea to think of the dry ice from science class.

Visual mnemonics come in all different forms. You can use words like "dog" for a dog's memory. You can use words like "world" for the world as a place. You can even use a blank picture and think about the scene or environment that it would create.

While there are many good mnemonics, they are not very good if you don't know how to use them properly. One of the easiest ways to remember a story or an event is to visualize it in your mind. This may work better if you do it before you say it or when saying it rather than after. For this reason, many people write down a few mnemonics on scrap pieces of paper or cards before going to sleep at night.

You can also use mnemonics in a business setting. For example, you might want to remind people that they have ten minutes to solve a problem, call a supervisor, or meet someone for lunch. You can draw a visual version of the problem or concern and use it as a time management tool. It can also help people relax or feel more comfortable doing a task. Just making the job more pleasant can help make it easier and faster to complete.

There are plenty of ways to write down mnemonics. One popular method is to write down everything you can think of about a specific subject or situation. Then, figure out which pieces of information will best describe that subject. Once you have done this, write a new story about what you have just discovered. You can even include pictures of what you have seen.

Mnemonics are great in a sports setting. If you are leading a winning race, you can mentally walk yourself through the finish line. Think about how you felt as you crossed the finish line. Think about how good it feels to win and how excited you will be when you next run.

Visual mnemonics are used in education settings a lot as well. For example, teachers can picture a student in a lesson and draw how that student might behave under certain conditions. This helps the teacher demonstrate how certain behaviors will be beneficial under certain conditions. They can then show people real-life examples of how these behaviors would be helpful. Visual stories and pictures can help people think more clearly.

# How to use mnemonic techniques

How to use Mnemonic techniques for memory improvement is a question that is asked by many. The answer depends on the person's personal situation and habits. If you are like most people, your answer is probably "I use them all the time." You might not be aware of it but your memory plays an important role in your everyday life. It can be helpful to review some basics about memory improvement such as what it is and why you need it. Then you can ask yourself:

What is Memory? Memory is the process by which we retain information. This includes how we remember names, facts, dates, emotions and other objects. When we can effortlessly recall these memories, we feel that we are in a better position to handle things.

Mnemonic techniques for memory improvement use words that we frequently use in our daily lives. These words are then made into images that we can visualize in our minds and this helps in improving our memory. These techniques help to improve our ability to remember things and remember them faster. When you repeatedly see the same word or phrase, it starts to become a habit and you start to use it even when you do not have to require it.

So what are the most commonly used memory improvement techniques? For short term memory improvement, the most used technique is mnemonics. Mnemonics are pictures or images that you can use to help you remember things. There are lots of ways to do this; you can use stories, images, flashcards and so on.

As an example, if you want to improve your short-term memory, you might use a picture of a hammer followed by its related words. Or if you are studying finance, you can use the words credit and loan. If you are studying cooking, you can use butter, ingredients and so on. Remember to attach the word to the item that you are trying to remember. This way, it becomes more memorable and improves your chances of remembering it.

Another example would be mnemonics for long-term memory improvement. Let's say that you are a teacher. You want to improve your classroom management skills. One way of improving your classroom management skills would be to associate your students' grades with the activities that they do during class time. So for every five minutes of activity, you give a small reward or a sticker.

Mnemonic techniques for memory improvement techniques are also widely used in learning how to play chess. Students are taught to identify and remember the important ideas that they should remember to make the next move. This way, they do not forget those crucial notions which they have already learnt - the important chess ideas.

How to use these techniques is simple. Just remember the important notions that you are supposed to remember and associate them with other words that you know. Soon enough, you will have improved your memory.

Mnemonic techniques for memory improvement techniques also help people in mastering the art of goal setting. When you set goals, you always have a number that you aim to achieve. However, when it comes to goal setting, there are a lot of things that you have to consider. First is the goal itself; then, you have to consider the obstacles that you need to overcome and finally, you have to come up with strategies on how you can make your goal achievable.

Through memorization, you strengthen your brain and at the same time, it improves your brain's function. For example, if you want to be an effective leader, you have to remind yourself of the things that you have done well whenever you think about being a leader. This method is called goal memorization. By doing so, you train your brain to work efficiently and you strengthen your memorization skill.

Mnemonic techniques for memory improvement techniques can also be learned through audio programs. These programs are specially designed to teach people about the importance of memory and how to improve memory. Aside from helping you remember things, these programs also promote brain fitness. They improve your cognitive functions and in the end, you will feel more confident. So, start training your brain using audio programs by downloading them from the internet.

Mnemonic techniques for memory improvement techniques are considered to be one of the best ways in improving your memory. It is not only a technique that you can use for a short period of time; it is also one that you can use for a long period of time. As such, if you really want to improve your memory, learn these simple methods today.

# Chapter 2

## Unconventional Studying Techniques

Unconventional Studying Techniques abound, even in the 21st century. Students are no longer confined to the traditional learning experience with books and lectures. These days, they can choose to get their learning done through the computer, using multimedia tutorials, or by joining online learning institutions that offer learning experiences tailored for individual needs. All of these methods offer advantages and disadvantages, and the learners must determine which ones suit them best.

Technology has been changing the way we study ever since the invention of the computer. This has been accompanied by the growth of unconventional methods such as distance learning and online courses. With these newer options available, does one still have to stick to the traditional method of studying? The answer depends on a few factors. While technology continues to advance, students can still choose the method that offers them the most convenience.

Time is still the biggest factor in traditional learning. Since students cannot be with their classmates at every hour of the day, it makes sense to stick to a schedule.
However, this doesn't always work out. Some students are tied up with jobs and cannot spend hours on campus to study; thus, they are left with few options but to learn unconventionally via the computer, on their free time.

Online Studying techniques are gaining popularity, because they allow students to study at their own pace, and at any time of the day or night. Students can take care of the class requirements and do other things while going to and from school. There is no need to be available to attend scheduled classes. This flexibility benefits students the most, and gives them more time to enjoy other activities.

Studying in groups is also more time-convenient than studying unmonitored by one instructor. In large classes, it is not uncommon for multiple instructors to give different instructions at the same time, making it difficult for students to retain information or to work on their assignments. With group studying, students are able to work on a problem together, and they get the help they need from one instructor.

As mentioned above, it is important to choose a learning style that fits your personal needs. Not all students are comfortable with group learning. If you need a traditional, one-on-one learning environment, then you should go to an onsite campus that offers traditional classrooms. For some students, even having the chance to meet their professors in person is not enough to satisfy their need for self-led learning.

Studying online has many advantages over traditional campus learning. For one, distance education allows students to work at their own pace. This means that they can put off some classes or materials for a later time. The material they learn can be reviewed whenever it is convenient for them. Online unconventional studwork can also be copied and distributed to other students, further increasing its convenience.

Studying online is an effective choice for many students. If you have a hectic schedule, however, you may want to consider going to a traditional campus. If you would rather keep things private, you can meet with your fellow students on a virtual forum. Either way, there are plenty of benefits to be had by learning online.

In order to successfully pursue unconventional learning, one must remember that studying does not always come easy. Sometimes, students have to exert a great deal of effort just to get through a class. However, the rewards of the work are well worth it. You will gain valuable knowledge, develop skills, and prepare yourself for a career. All of these things are important to consider if you are planning to pursue this degree.

Before you start studying, it is important for you to think about how long you plan to study for. While it is not necessary to complete your studies in a set number of years, you should make sure to make this a priority. If you are not able to commit to a certain amount of time, then you should consider finding a roommate or finding an online school that allows you to share your space. This will allow you to take care of your own studies and help you to stay on track.

Remember, an unconventional stud does not necessarily mean that they have low self-esteem. Many people are extremely gifted academically but choose to pursue careers in fields that do not emphasize their abilities. If you are interested in learning more about this type of field, consider seeking out unconventional learning opportunities. There are many different programs available so you should not feel limited by your resources. You can pursue a successful education!

If you're tired of studying the same old textbook on boring subjects that never seem to be interesting enough to make you remember what you learned, then Unconventional Studying Techniques might just be for you. Studying in an irregular time-frame is one of the easiest and most effective ways to boost your memory and comprehension scores. If you're like most people who can't schedule themselves to study for a regular class, then this method of learning may be just what you need.

The concept is simple. Instead of studying for sets amounts of time during the day, try studying unconventionalistically for fifteen minutes each day. You can easily do this with Unconventional Studying Techniques by recording what you are doing on a notebook or text file as you go. You can then go back and review anything that seemed to be unclear before falling asleep. If you have time, try studying unconventionalistically for up to thirty minutes at a time.

What makes Unconventional Studying Techniques so effective? The key to it is making sure that the brain doesn't become tired from constant study. It's easy to become unfocused after spending several hours staring at a computer screen. Studies show that when the brain isn't constantly exposed to a certain material, it can have a hard time focusing and can even damage brain cells.

When the brain is exposed to a constant flow of new materials, it is able to focus better and remember better. This also makes Unconventional Studying Techniques a valuable addition to any student's toolbox. It has worked for many students, including myself, as it allows me to learn new material in less time while having fun doing so. After a few months of practicing, I found that I was able to retain information from materials longer than usual. Now, I don't study for an hour or more in most days, but I always find time to study for at least fifteen minutes or so.

Another Unconventional Studying Techniques that have worked well for me is to keep a visual reminder in my head of the material I am studying. For me, this would be a piece of paper with the required information printed on it. I would read it over in my mind each night before bed. When I get up in the morning, I can mentally review what I learned during the day. This habit has paid off big for me as I have been able to increase my grade point average by several grades because I always remember what I learned during the day.

Studying in the middle of the night might not sound very practical, but for some people it can prove to be very helpful. You may find it helpful to study in your bedroom, on your night off, or any other place that you feel comfortable. Your brain is just as powerful as it is while you are sleeping, so why shouldn't it be working while you are studying?

Unconventional Studying Techniques such as these will work for you if you are willing to give them a shot. I urge you to give them a try, but don't expect results immediately. Studying is an ever-evolving field and there is always more that people are learning. Just keep at it. Over time, maybe some of these Unconventional Studying Techniques will become much more effective for you.

Studying is a great experience, but some students don't like studying in a quiet dark room. If this describes you, consider using one or more of the Unconventional Studying Techniques mentioned above. Don't give up. Studying isn't easy and you need to push yourself to excel at it. Sometimes, all you need is an extra push.

Unconventional Studying Techniques can make a big difference in your learning experience. Studying in the way that is most effective for you, however, may not always match up to what your textbook or instructor tells you to do. Some students are naturally visual while others need to learn more by listening and really absorbing the information. It's important to be flexible in how you learn and adapt your studies to suit the lesson.

You should never feel limited or pressured into a certain method of studying. Your personal style should guide your learning approach as well as your level of comprehension. Listen to the song or artist and then play it back so that you can hear how the melody works with the rhythm. If you can do this, you have a solid foundation for understanding the song.

When you listen to an unconventional song, focus on what it does better than what you are usually taught. For instance, listen to how each verse changes up the song. This will give you a different perspective on the song than what your instructor may be telling you. Think out of the box and see how the song could have been played otherwise.

Don't try to memorize all the notes and guitar chords. Try to visualize the song. Instead of trying to memorize every note and chord, try to visualize each movement of the hands. By doing so, you will be able to play the song in your mind much faster. If you can envision the song, it will become easier to learn how to play it.

Unconventional Studying Techniques can make a big difference in your learning.
Try not to get too caught up in theory. It's fine to have some knowledge in the subject but there are plenty of ways of putting it to use by applying it to a real situation. Instead of reading the definition of a word, why not see how it can be used in context with the lyrics or the song?

Don't be afraid to improvise when studying music. Sometimes playing around with something in the right key and tempo can yield amazing results. You might think that practicing scales is an easy way to learn new songs, but it's something else entirely. Improvisation should be at the forefront of your studies, instead of waiting for theory to catch up to your ears. Studying unconventional methods to learn music will take you places.

Studying in a group is another great way to learn something. When you get a group of students to study together, you get more individual attention. Some students get too used to studying in their own private homes and forget about the importance of group study. Learning in a group environment boosts your self-esteem and makes you a more rounded student. If you are unable to find a study partner, consider joining a study group.

The last tip I have for you in regard to unconventional Studying is to ignore personal opinion when making a decision. It's easy to say that your favorite class is great, but what if the professor is the worst? Your best friend probably dislikes the class you are taking and would never recommend it to anyone else. So don't get wrapped up in your own experiences and opinions when choosing to pursue a course or college.

A good way to get out of the typical groove is to visit a number of campuses during your Studying Year. Get to know the campus and find the ambiance that best suits you. You may also want to see how the students in your class interact with each other. When visiting a campus, make sure to pay attention to the unusual things you notice. It's possible that you will meet an unconventional stud who has overcome the typical hurdles in studying.

There is no better way to start to study than by immersing yourself in a new environment. Immersion Studying allows you to become immersed in a new culture and learn firsthand from its people. The more you get to know your fellow students, the easier it will be for you to adjust to their way of life. It is easier to adapt to an unconventional stud's way of life, than it would be sitting in a classroom surrounded by traditional students.

Immersion Studying allows you to gain a unique understanding about what life is like on your chosen campus. When you become accustomed to a college's culture, you will begin to see the most important aspects of that culture. You will begin to see the people in everyday life, and how they react to situations. Studying in an unconventional environment makes it easier to pick up the language and culture of that country. Immersion Studying is definitely a great way to increase your knowledge of the campus you are going to, and it is also a great way to discover unique individuals who are a part of that campus.

# Chapter 3

## Mnemonic deals with the information and methods
## What are the mnemonic methods?

What are the mnemonic methods? For those who don't know, a mnemonic is a memory trick that helps you find something you're looking for. For example, if you're searching for an address, you would use the words of an address such as "attle rattle barn", which would help you remember it. A good mnemonic trick can help you to remember any kind of thing. There's no limit to the things you can train yourself to remember. With a little practice, and a lot of patience, the mnemonic methods will come to you easily.

How can mnemonic methods help you? It all comes down to your mind being able to focus on a single idea. For some people this is very easy, especially if they already have an idea in their heads. For others, especially those who aren't so talented, this is a bit harder to achieve. It helps to keep a mental picture of the object you want to memorize.

So how do you use mnemonics to remember anything? You find a good book that has an image you like to repeat. If you can focus on the image for a long enough period of time, you will be able to recall it. Nowadays, books are designed to be extremely easy to read. So you won't even have to strain your eyes trying to find anything.

If you can concentrate hard enough to remember a list of phone numbers, you can find anything anywhere. You could go through every phone book and count all the numbers. If you want to remember them, it's okay to write them down and then look at them whenever you need a mental image. This technique is a lot more effective than trying to find anything anywhere else.

The next step up from mnemonic methods is to learn about memory tricks. This means learning about the visual associations we have with things. So if we have the mnemonic to remember the number 6, wouldn't it be easier to link that to something else? So instead of saying get the beer pot, instead link it to something else like the beach.

If you're interested in learning a mnemonic, there is a long and fascinating history to it. The Chinese developed a mnemonic method that helped them to remember more. In fact, they used pictorial representations in order to remember information. Romans also developed a similar system using coins that represented money and dates that represented time. When studying the histories of these ancient people, you might find that they were actually using more than just mnemonic methods. They were actually using lots of different methods of remembering, but they needed to remember each one separately.

The question of what are the mnemonic methods? was important in studying the development of language and how memory works. Not only can we remember words, but we can also remember entire paragraphs, ideas, or whole pieces of song lyrics. Even the process of putting a puzzle together is not a simple task without a mental image of the solution. It's as if we're trying to piece together a jigsaw puzzle that just doesn't fit right.

Although we know that our brains are extremely powerful machines, there are limits. We can only think so fast, and we can only remember so much. Even with mnemonic tools such as flashcards or index cards, we won't remember everything the first time we see it. So although those mnemonic methods are fun, they may not give you the greatest results in the end.

The good news is that by using something like an index card or a flashcard, you can memorize much faster than you could by using a pen and paper. The reason why it's faster to write things down is because you have to use your fingers for control. With just a glance, you are able to move from one word to the next. This gives you the opportunity to evaluate which mnemonic method will work best for you in your studies.

Even though there are various methods of mnemonics, using one of them will not get you the results you want. You have to adapt it to suit you. If you study vocabulary in a different way, it won't help you memorize more easily. Similarly, if you focus on the rhyme, then it may take longer for you to remember than those who choose other methods. The most important thing is to find the best combination for you so you can memorize much faster and easier.

Another option that you can explore is finding websites that offer their own unique mnemonics. There are some sites that give you the option to try their "favorites" and "secret techniques". These online favorites and secrets can help you memorize much faster as well. You will even get to find out what other people prefer using for mnemonics. You may also get to learn how others are using certain mnemonics for a particular task. Such information can be extremely useful in your studies.

# What are the 3 main components of mnemonics?

Mnemonics have been used for years to aid memory development. There are many different ways to use mnemonics, but it is mainly because they are so effective that they have been incorporated into many different learning strategies. They can also be used in place of lists or graphs, to make a new learning activity more interesting and effective. Here are the three main components of mnemonics, along with some examples of how they can be used.

The first component is the words that are used in the mnemonic. While you would have to come up with a pretty good list of words to use in a mnemonic, it is a good idea to include at least some of the most common words that students might use. This is because the words would be used often, and would therefore be memorized quite quickly. For example, the first two elements in a shopping list might be "shopping", and "list".

The second main element of a good mnemonic would be the main body of text. This could be an essay, an outline, an explanation, or even just a few sentences. What is important is that this text should focus on the main elements that are needed for the item to stand out from all others. For example, if a list is being used in a shopping memory game, the text that is used should focus on the list, and not the products that are listed. It is also okay to add in some personal information about the list as well.

The third and final component of a good mnemonic is the images that are used in the mnemonic. Again, this would need to be something that is important enough to use in the short term, but that would change over time so that the mind does not become too attached to any one image. It can be a simple picture, or it can be something more complex, such as a photograph or a drawing.

If you take all three elements and use them in any mnemonic, you will end up with a fairly accurate description. This is what are the 3 main components of mnemonics. They are the main body of the text, the pictures that will be used in the text, and the way that they will be remembered after the initial use. When you start to teach yourself how to use mnemonics, these are the three things that you will need to focus on.

The main body of the text is the main part of the message itself. This could be information that someone passes along to you, or it could be information that you have to process in order to use mnemonics in your own learning. Regardless of how it comes across to you, it needs to be a short sentence or two long. The more simple the better. Just think about all the times when you have heard the word "Mary" and you associated that with cooking, gardening, or some other related activity.

After you have your main text, you will need a bunch of images or pictures that will be used in the text. The pictures can be quite varied and can be anything from simple photographs to paintings or even computer generated images. Just make sure that they will be able to be easily read when the mnemonic is being used. You will also want to include a few verbs or words that will be repeated throughout the message. Again, the more you use the word, the easier they will be to remember and use in the writing.

Now that you know the answer to "what are the 3 main components of mnemonics?" you can begin to actually use mnemonics in your own teaching. When you are teaching an introduction to language class, it is very helpful if you can relate the text to something that students already know or care about. Even if they do not, it is still important for them to be able to remember it. Even if they do not understand what is being illustrated, using a good mnemonic will help them to remember it later. And hopefully they will eventually be able to explain it to you!

# What are mnemonics used for?

When people hear the word "mnemonic" they get a feeling of vague familiarity. Perhaps they've heard it somewhere before but can't quite pinpoint where or when it came from. It can mean the difference between a good study session and a terrible one. You wouldn't want your students memorizing the last five lyrics to Seal or The Who's "I Remember You." Or how about the nursery rhymes "Goodnight, Sleep Tight, and Good Morning," which can make even the most tranquil of sleep disorders sound like an ordeal.

So what are mnemonics? In simple terms, they are mental pictures or images that help you keep track of time and information. They are an essential tool for the memorization process. There are a wide variety of mnemonics and learning techniques available.

You may have heard that mnemonics are nothing more than "memory aids." That's true up to a point. The usefulness of a memory aid is limited by the ability of the individual to remember what was initially visualized. An image or word does not mean anything unless it is able to be recalled and then remembered by the individual.

When you read out loud or hear your own voice you may instantaneously be able to "hear" the words or phrases. When you read or hear a sentence aloud, you have to take time to mentally re-read what was just said. This is where the usefulness of mnemonics comes in.

In many cases, a writer or speaker will use a series of words or phrases to "anchor" a paragraph, an entire essay, or a section of a presentation. These anchoring words or phrases are generally embedded in a lengthy explanation of some sort. The intent is to make the reader understand that the entire statement is worth reading and thinking about. The embedded words or phrases are then used as a reminder of the main point or thesis of the essay or other piece of literature. For example, if a writer is talking about cancer and he mentions a specific disease that is part of cancer, he may use the word cancer mnemonics in order to remind the audience that the disease should be taken seriously.

So what are mnemonics used for? They are commonly used in courses in English grammar, composition, and writing. Usually a teacher will present her students with a list of words, phrases, or sentences that will help them study a passage and analyze its various elements. Then, as the class progresses, the students are asked to identify which parts of the passage were most useful in helping them construct their own opinions and arguments about the passage.

So what are mnemonics used for? One reason why they are so helpful is because they force students to pay close attention to the exact wording and structure of the passage. This kind of close attention helps students analyze and compare the different arguments that are presented in order to come up with their own opinions and statements about the matter at hand. It also forces students to think about the best ways to say or write the particular phrase or word that was chosen. After all, the purpose of using mnemonics is not just to memorize words but to convince the reader that one's arguments are the most sensible.

What are mnemonics used for? It really depends on who is asking, but the most common reason why teachers use mnemonics in teaching is because they help students remember the main points and themes of a lesson. They serve as excellent guideposts and constant reminders of what things should be written or read. In short, a good example of a mnemonic is the famous quote "A teacher can have many students, but only a few students will use it."

# Chapter 4

## Learn The Mnemonics

Do you want to learn the Mnematics for High School Students? This is something that many high school students struggle with, especially when they are starting to learn the language. Learning a second language is never easy and there is a lot of work that goes into turning something into a memorized form. When it comes to the Mnematics for High School Students, there are some tricks that can be used to make sure that memory is made easier. These mnemonics will help to bring more focus to words and sentences that have already been learned so that you can have better success with finding the translations of the words.

There are several good sources for learning the most effective mnemonics and one of the best ways is to use flash cards that have Mnemonics as an example of the topics being covered. How do you help high year 2 students to remember the foreign spellings of medical terms? By using these great mnemonic poster display boards. Learn the various mnemonics with these handy mnemonic posters and then display them in your class.

Using mnemonics is not just limited to flash cards. You can also find various types of paper mnemonics that are just placed on a certain page or board. These are great for students that like to write and try to memorize everything that they see. Another great source for these mnemographs is by using controlled practice tests. These kinds of test-taking strategies will give students real life scenarios to think about when they are memorizing phrases. They can work hard at developing their memory skills and still get a decent test grade because they are working under controlled conditions.

Learn the nitty gritty details of these kinds of mnemics by downloading a Learn The Mnemonics eBook from my website. This is a very easy to read eBook that is full of both practical and proven tactics to help students learn and memorize more effectively. This is a must have for any student that wants to go beyond good grades in school. If you are serious about getting better grades, then you need to make sure that you are using these memorization aids.

Learn the various nitty gritty details of these types of memory aids by downloading Learn The Mnemonics eBook online. This is a must have for any student that wants to go beyond good grades in school. If you are serious about getting better grades, then you need to make sure that you are using these memorization aids.

One of the best World War II novels ever written, "The World War II" by H. G. Wells is considered one of the top books on the list. It is considered a classic that harkens back to the days of World War II. Students who study World War II must make sure that they read this excellent novel. In addition to the rich colorful plot of the story, the characters are very relatable, which makes this book a favorite among many people.

Students who are planning on taking exams for higher education purposes should definitely make time to read this text. Students who are preparing for test can greatly benefit from this book as well.
This is a rich description of many historic battles. Reading this text will enlighten students on just how the soldiers on both sides suffered from such difficulties.

The author, Wells, did an excellent job of describing the suffering both sides endured during World War II. Reading through the book, students can see exactly what the soldiers had to go through. They can also learn about the things that they had to carry with them while fighting. Students can learn the significance of the pocket watches that the military used as they marched around.

Students can use the knowledge learned from this text in many aspects of their lives. Learning the Mnemonics can be used to help students get better grades in school. This book can be used as a reference when writing test and exam papers. Students can also use it when writing essays and even in conversation. When creating a resume, a student can make sure that he or she includes the appropriate mnemonics. This can be done before submitting the resume to ensure that the resume stands out from the rest of the crowd.

The use of mnemonics in many different aspects of life can help students succeed in life. When learning the Mnemonics, students should make sure to study the lessons in an organized manner. They should use the knowledge learned from the text not in isolation but in conjunction with other things that they already know. The use of mnemonics should be remembered and used properly in order for students to reach their full educational potential.

# Chapter 5

## NCLEX Exam

The National Council Licensure Examination (NCLEX) is a nationally recognized test for the licensure of medical nurses in the United States, Canada, Australia and New Zealand since 1981. It is compulsory for all aspiring nurses to take the exam so that they can be eligible for a nursing practice. There are two versions, the NCLEX -RN and NCLEX -PN. The NCLEX -RN is the entry-level examination, whereas the NCLEX -PN is the higher-level examination.

The passing standard for this exam is 80%. However, there are a number of steps and study tips available for successful completion of the NCLEX. For starters, all students should select a qualified instructor. Some of the well-known nursing institutions offer NCLEX coaching programs. These help students to prepare properly before the examination.

They provide sample questions and answers and study strategies which can greatly help in preparing for the NCLEX. Students can also check the official results of the last three years and find out their pass rates. The official results of the six weeks preceding the exam helps in deciding on the pass rates.

After determining the pass rates, students should submit their application to the state board.
However, there are certain rules and regulations that must be followed by each student. Firstly, they should seek permission to sit for the NCLEX. Then they should undergo training for nursing. In case of non-compliance, they may be disqualified from sitting for the NCLEX.

Each state board requires applicants to submit proof of training or examination to show that they possess the minimum number of credit hours as required by them. However, applicants should ensure that they get informed about the passing rates before applying. Students have to pay a fee to the state board. Some colleges also charge fees for NCLEX practice tests.

Apart from that, applicants should allot five hours of quiet time before and after the test.

For students who want to be able to pass the NCLEX without much trouble, they should choose the tests that are available online. This ensures that they practice enough to become familiar with the types of questions asked. They should also have adequate time allocated for studying.

Applicants can contact the regulatory board for assistance in preparing for NCLEX exams. It will help in ensuring that they do not spend too much time in reviewing the contents of the NCLEX. The regulatory board also provides sample questions and answers. Applicants should make sure that they understand the meaning of the terms in the text books and the meaning of the diagrams in the exams.

In order to reduce the time spent on the examination, students should allot a certain number of hours for preparation. Applicants should seek advice from friends and nursing educators to know how to prepare for NCLEX examinations. They should also study for two to four weeks before the examination. They can also apply for NCLEX study guide to give them an idea on the various subjects that they will be required to study.

Students need to be familiar with the computerized design format of the NCLEX examination. This is required because the examination includes questions that are based on information provided by computerized systems. The exam measures a nurses' capability to analyze health data. This is important because medical research shows that human beings are less able to analyze health data compared to those that are provided by computers. Computerized systems for answering NCLEX examinations have gained more popularity among applicants in recent years.

Students should look into their exam appointment prior to the exam day. They should discuss with their faculty who will give the exam. The exam schedule will be published three weeks prior to the exam date. Nursing educators are the best source of information on NCLEX exam schedule. They can provide information on exam registration, fee structures, exam fees, and NCLEX study materials.

There are two types of NCLEX study guides that are designed to help nursing candidates prepare for the NCLEX. The first type is hands-on practice by using real exam questions from the NCLEX. The second type of study guide is a study guide that contains a complete list of all of the questions that will appear on the NCLEX. Both types of study guides are very valuable and useful to nursing candidates who want to excel in the NCLEX.

The NCLEX is a test that requires both knowledge and skill. Candidates need to review and learn a lot about the subjects that they will be tested on. During the preparation process, they should engage in practicing the skills that they plan to use on the NCLEX. The best way to study for the NCLEX is through taking computer adaptive testing exams. These exams are available online and can be downloaded to a student's computer so that they can do practice exams whenever they want.

# What does the NCLEX exam consist of?

The NCLEX is the examination that must be taken in order to be able to take the NCLEX-RN test. This test is required by all nurses who want to take their practice tests again. This means that it is the most important exam in the nursing career. It is a combination of theory and skills, and when you take the proper preparations you will do well on the NCLEX exam.

Before you even start studying for the exam, make sure that you have a list of questions that you need to study. This can help you determine which books are best to buy. The reason why you want to buy the right books is because you will want to get ones that are formatted correctly so that you do not have any problems when you sit down to take the actual test. Make sure that you take the time to review your books before you even begin studying.

One of the most important tools that you will need is a NCLEX study guide. There are a number of them that you can purchase from various bookstores or even online. Some of them like The Nifty Company have very thorough and organized guides that allow you to get an overview of the test. If you feel like you are being challenged, then this type of guide could really come in handy.

You will also want to have at least three months before the test a full analysis of what has happened in your career. Think about what has happened in each of the two year periods leading up to your test. How have you managed to maintain your career, what changes have you made, and what are your plans for the future? This will give you an idea of how you will fare on the test.

Now that you are prepared, the next step in what does the NCLEX exam consist of? The next step is practice tests. You must do plenty of practice tests to familiarize yourself with all of the different types of questions that you will be faced with. You can buy NCLEX practice tests online or you can bring a printed copy of any of the tests you took in high school to your local testing center. Make sure that you take plenty of time for this part of the preparation.

Now that you have some understanding of what to expect when taking the test, it's time to start studying for the test. You should definitely spend at least a couple of hours every single day studying. Don't try to study on your own during this time because you may make a wrong assumption that will cost you points. Instead, set up a system where you study for the NCLEX ahead of time and then stick to it. By doing so, you will know when your time is right to take the actual exam.

Now that you have prepared yourself for the test, it's time to start practicing. Again, don't try to study too much before your test, just take small, quick notes while doing so. Practice makes perfect, especially with this one because you won't have any questions to actually answer during the test. When practicing, it's important that you don't pace yourself, otherwise you will end up being tired and not focused during the test. Instead, just focus on taking small notes every few minutes until you feel that you are ready to start taking the actual NCLEX.

Once you get through answering all of the questions posed, you will be given a score. This is the final exam grade, so you want to make sure you get a good mark here. This is why it's so important that you go over everything thoroughly. After you have gone over the material, take a few practice tests to make sure you have covered all the things you need to know. As long as you've studied, cleaned up your schedule, practiced, and taken a test or two, you should be well on your way to an easy and successful NCLEX exam!

# Is the NCLEX hard to pass?

Is the NCLEX hard to pass? If you've gone through the testing process once and passed, that's great! However, if you failed it a second time you might be asking yourself if you can pass the NCLEX for the third time and not have to spend another three years earning an RN degree before getting your license. There are many who have been able to do so. The question is how did they do it and what can you do to ensure that you pass it the next time around?

Good signs that you have passed the NCLEX is if you no longer have to take any further nursing classes. Failing the NCLEX isn't the end of the world though. In fact, many RNs just completed their third or fourth time trying to get into a specific specialty. This means that they have spent a lot of time and money to achieve their goal. You should feel good about achieving your goal and taking it to the next level.

It is always a good idea to review before taking the test. The NCLEX is a complex test that deals with theory and practical aspects of nursing. As such, it is a good idea to read as much as you can about the test and your specific areas of focus. This will allow you to have a greater understanding of what you will be expected to do during the actual test. Don't skimp on this part of the preparation. It's essential to do.

Another important aspect of preparing for the test is making sure you get plenty of rest. This isn't just about sleep though. Rest can help you to relax and refresh yourself before the test. Too much stress and fatigue can throw off your concentration on the NCLEX.

If you are having trouble with the NCLEX, don't beat yourself up too much. There are several reasons why someone might be having a hard time passing the NCLEX. Most often it has more to do with them than it has to do with the test itself. Perhaps they simply weren't practicing their breathing and relaxation techniques. The best way to find out why you aren't doing well is to take the time to find out why you aren't doing as well as you could.

If the reason you aren't as effective at the NCLEX as you'd like is because you simply aren't practicing enough, then consider taking a practice test or two before the real test. Don't worry if the first one you take does not go well. Try the next one. There is no such thing as failure when it comes to the NCLEX. Eventually you will get better at taking tests and performing under pressure.

Another common reason that people give is that they are taking the test because they want to get certification. Although this is an important goal, if that's your only motivation, then you will likely fail. There are plenty of students who are also motivated by the benefits of being certified. If you can stay motivated and focused on those benefits, then you will succeed.

The answer to the question is the NCLEX hard to pass? should be "not as hard." If you are motivated, knowledgeable, and prepared, then you have a good chance of passing. So don't lose hope if you've had a history of bad scores on this test before.

Now, it's important to remember that if you really want to take this exam, you need to invest in some study guides. These are typically sold separately or as part of an online course. They typically contain sample questions and tips for every section, and will help you get ready for the big day. If you want to get the most out of studying for this test, then these are your best option.

Is the NCLEX hard to pass? should be "no." By doing all of the tips and practice questions in these guides, you will have no problem passing the NCLEX. Just be sure that you are committed to learning and taking action, instead of just sitting back and expecting the answer to come to you.

Want to learn how to increase your chances of getting the top NCLEX points possible? Get my latest eBook and start improving your score today! This eBook is full of useful information for effectively mastering the NCLEX.

# 6 Things to Know About the NCLEX Exam

The NCLEX is an important test that is required for those aspiring nurses. This exam is considered to be the most difficult exam in all of nursing. This is because it test both your logic and critical thinking skills. If you are planning to take this exam, then the first thing you need to do is find a study guide that will help you prepare for it. Not all study guides are made equal.

The study guide should be able to teach you all the information that you will need during the test and at the same time it should cover all the types of questions that can appear on the exam. You should also be able to figure out how to use the various tools that are available during the test. Most people spend thousands of dollars on this exam, so you need to make sure that you get the best possible preparation before taking the test. There are a few tips that will help you with finding the best study guide.

The first thing you need to do is find reviews of NCLEX study guides. These reviews are widely available on the internet and they will tell you which ones are good and which ones are useless. The more reviews you read, the better. The next step you should do is figure out which study guides are going to help you the most. To do this, you should consider the amount of time you have to study.

The review material that is available should include practice tests. The NCLEX has two different tests that are taken, the practical and the verbal. The practice test is going to give you a better idea about what you are going to face during the actual test. Some review material will tell you about how to deal with certain obstacles on the exam, but not much.

Once you have a list of questions that you think you can answer accurately, it's time to take the practice test. This can be quite tricky because if you start it too early, you may find it hard to remember all of the questions. If you can take the test early, then make sure that you start reviewing when you start feeling tired. Try to study for two hours before taking the actual test. Make sure that you have your study materials or they won't help you remember what you read.

Once you've done the practice test, it's time to review the information that you read and to prepare for the real test. Review material will include anything that covered in the practice test. You want to make sure that all of the topics were covered so you know what to expect. By the time you take the real test, you should know exactly what to expect.

If you take the time to learn about how the NCLEX works, then you are going to find it much easier to pass the exam. It is not going to be easy, but it can be done. If you don't take the time to study, then the only way that you will improve is if you get the study guide. These study guides will allow you to review everything you want to about the NCLEX.

In order to make sure that you don't have any misconceptions about the NCLEX, you need to read this article. We hope that you learned something new about the NCLEX and that you are now ready to take the real exam. It's important to review the material in this article and to get as much information as possible about the NCLEX. Once you have learned all that you can about the NCLEX, you can take the practice tests and make sure that you really understand what is going to happen on the day of the exam.

# Breaking the ice for nclex exam

When I took the NCLEX in 2021, I had no idea what to expect. I had heard so many people talk about taking the exam and I had visions of being able to write an essay or two and pass with flying colors. Well, let me tell you that I was way ahead of the curve and received some outstanding grades on my exams. So now I am here to share with you some tips and tricks that will really help you when it comes to answering the NCLEX. First of all, before you even start your research, you need to know what the NCLEX is all about. If you have no idea what that is then do some research and find out.

The NCLEX is a nationally recognized standardized exam that is designed to test your reading, writing, speaking, and listening skills. It is a very difficult test and you only get one try before the results are in. You will likely be asked to come in at least four times and take the test. This can become rather stressful, but if you are prepared it can really help you. One of the best ways you can prepare for this exam is to meet with a tutor. If you can meet with a tutor for an entire four hours before the exam then it will really be helpful.

You should also make sure that you have all of the materials you need beforehand and have reviewed them. This will help you to relax during the exam and it will also make it easier for you to remember what you read. You will be doing so many multiple-choice questions so you need to make sure that you have studied everything ahead of time.

You also want to create a mindset before the exam. Make sure that you have a positive frame of mind. Many people who try to study too much before the exam often experience a negative response from the test. This is something that you do not want to happen.

Most people who prepare well for exams are able to pass them with flying colors. However, for those that don't there are steps you can take to help you do well on the exam. You don't want to feel anxious or fear driven. Being too nervous about taking an exam is just going to make you have a bad time. This may not be a life-threatening exam, but it is a test that requires some skill.

There are things you should be aware of when it comes to taking an official test like the NCLEX. One of the things that can help you when it comes to breaking the ice for the NCLEX exam is proper timing. You want to find the best way to approach the exam and this involves proper scheduling. If you don't get the proper amount of sleep then you won't be as prepared as you could be.

Another key to success is having a positive attitude. Many people get very negative when they think about exams. They want to end up on the wrong side of the exam. However, this will not help you at all. You want to be as positive as possible and try to look at the exam in the best light.

When you are approaching the exam make sure to have a few open conversations. When you sit down with your friends and family talk about what you can expect coming into the exam room. Everyone has different experiences with this is why you want to hear what others have gone through. You should never be too harsh on yourself or question how much you can do. By having a positive attitude, you will be prepared and ready to ace the NCLEX.

# Chapter 6

## What are the basics of pharmacology?

What are the essentials of pharmology? There are numerous schools of thought about what are the essentials of pharmology. Many people think that they know what pharmology is, but often they are only half right. This article will address what are the essentials of pharmology to the extent that they are relevant to the practice of modern pharmacology. What are the essentials of pharmacology?

The essentials of pharmacology comprise of 4 main elements; biology, chemistry, mathematics and anatomy. These are the parts of pharmacology, although it should be noted that pharmacology can also encompass other disciplines such as psychology, radiology, and other medical subjects. In any event, these four main elements form the basis for the study of pharmacology.

The study of these four elements should give rise to what are the essentials of pharmacology. To begin with, biology is the first element in what are the essentials of pharmology? Biology addresses everything from understanding the function of microorganisms to the nature of detoxification processes. This study will include both the structure and function of molecules and cells as well as the functions of hormones, enzymes, and transporters.

Chemistry addresses the chemical makeup of different types of cells, tissues, organs, and metabolic processes. In addition, chemistry studies the interactions between chemicals. An example of a study would be studying pharmacological effects on enzyme actions in cells, which in turn affect different types of chemical reactions. This type of study may prove to be extremely useful in finding new medications that have effect on cells other than those affected by the pharmacological process itself.

Pharmacology also studies the distribution of chemicals in cells, organ systems, and the body. The study of how these chemicals act on target cells can prove to be extremely important in the development of new drugs. This type of study may even point to future treatments. Therefore, a pharmaceutical graduate student must be prepared to learn all of the essential elements of pharmacology.

Another key aspect of what are the essentials of pharmology? Learning about the development and balance of chemicals is another fundamental aspect that students must master if they wish to succeed in a career in this field. A comprehensive review of chemical composition is an essential part of the coursework for any graduate degree program in the field of pharmacology. In addition to this, students need to know when and how to balance chemicals in order to maximize their effects. Therefore, taking this course will prove to be one of the most essential elements of pharmology.

An understanding of cell structure is another crucial concept that students need to understand if they want to gain a successful understanding of what are the essentials of pharmology?
Cell structure is intimately connected to the function and structure of all cells within the body. Therefore, understanding cell function is vital to the study of pharmacology. The role of the micro-circulatory system in the function of a cell and the whole body is also an interesting area of study for students of this field. Thus, understanding the cell Structure connection is essential to developing an understanding of the what are the essentials of pharmology?

The concepts that are presented above are only a few of the many that will be encountered throughout a what are the essentials of pharmology? graduate program. Studying the basics of pharmacology in depth is an essential part of the Ph.D. program.

In addition to broad general studies, specific study in the areas of anatomy and physiology is an important part of the student's training. They should be given enough information to be able to understand the concepts presented above. Anatomy and physiology is very important to the field of medicine. Without the correct knowledge, it is impossible to diagnose and treat patients effectively. This is why students should be introduced to the concepts early in their career to ensure that they have the correct knowledge needed.

There are numerous ways to gain an understanding of what are the essentials of pharmology? Many students choose to take courses related to the essentials of pharmacology. This is usually best for those already in the field. It helps students to develop their knowledge as well as enhance their chances of finding a job after graduating. In addition to the coursework, students may choose to participate in clinical experiences or workshops to further increase their knowledge of pharmaceutical composition.

The knowledge of what are the essentials of pharmology? is necessary for every medical professional. Without a basic knowledge of the field, it would be difficult to learn the complexities of drug actions and how they affect the body. It is also important for doctors to be able to prescribe drugs with the correct dosage and proper concentration for maximum benefits to the patient. A general knowledge of pharmaceutical composition is essential for developing a solid foundation in pharmacology and eventually gaining positions of responsibility in hospitals, pharmaceutical companies, and other health care professions.

# How do I start learning pharmacology?

If you have ever asked yourself "How do I start learning pharmacology?" then I am sure that the answer will be very quick and straight forward for most people. There are a lot of people that get in a lot of trouble by not understanding the pharmaceutical sciences very well. This is because it is very hard to understand the pharmaceutical sciences if you do not have a lot of experience in them, so when someone asks you "How do I start learning pharmacology?"

So what most people tend to do when they want to start learning about any type of field is they try to get as much experience as they can and hopefully they will learn everything that they can possibly need to know in order to start out on their career in the pharmaceutical sciences.

This is a mistake that a lot of people make, but thankfully there is a way to avoid the mistakes that they normally do and that is through online courses. Online courses have become extremely popular recently, especially with online pharmacy schools and their growing demand for more college students to major in pharmacy majors. Online courses are a lot easier to take because you are taking the classes at home, in your own time, and you are not competing against a lot of other students that are trying to take the same classes as you.

The way that these online courses work is that you sign up for an online course from a pharmaceutical school or online pharmacy school. Once you have enrolled in that course you will receive all of the materials that you need to complete the required course. Then once the course is completed, you will be able to take a practice test from the school to see how far you have truly come. Online courses are extremely popular nowadays because it allows anyone to take the required courses from their own home, at their own pace and in the comfort of their own home. Many people will just take the class once in order to get their foot in the door, but this is not the way that you should go about starting your career in pharmaceuticals. So with that being said, if you want to start learning about pharmaceuticals, then online courses are your answer.

When you think of how to start learning about pharmacology, the first thing that probably comes to your mind is the pharmacy. This is definitely an important first step and one that many people take. However, it doesn't stop there; there are other aspects of this area that you need to become familiar with as well.

There are many different opportunities in the pharmaceutical field. You can get a job in research or do research in the lab. You can even work as a manager in a company doing everything from marketing to sales. If you want to learn about the entire field of pharmacology then you need to know about the different paths you can take to reach your goals.

One option that many people choose is to get a bachelor's degree. This will get you on your way towards a successful career in the medical field. Many employers look for candidates who have a higher level of education regardless of their career choice. If you want to start learning about this field then you will likely find that a bachelor's degree will get you on your way.

Once you graduate you can move forward in your career. It is possible to further your education and gain even more knowledge about this field. Your salary will depend greatly on where you go for your education. You may end up making a lot less money than someone who went to school for 4 years but also attended a prestigious university. You can also study online if you want to take advantage of some of the great programs offered today.

Even after you have some basic knowledge of pharmacology you may be interested in different fields. This is also a great option. There are so many different subjects you can study. You could become a veterinarian, anesthesiologist, pediatrician, etc. No matter what your interests are, you can pursue them.

You will also need to get the proper training for the positions you want to work in. You should have a bachelor's degree or higher in order to be eligible for many of the entry level jobs. You will also need to have relevant experience in your field. You should speak with a few different schools to see which one will offer you the best education. Depending on what type of work you want to do you may want to also consider any certificates or licensing you already have. You should also take into account any other training you have received.

In some cases a college degree will not be enough. In that case you will want to consider obtaining an Associate's degree. This will help you get the skills and knowledge you need for the job you are applying for. In many cases you will find that this is all you need to get the job you want.

When looking at how do I start learning about pharmacology? The first step is to get educated. There are many options for you to pursue in order to get the education you need. Once you are educated you can take the next step and begin your career in a pharmaceutical lab.

When you are trying to figure out how do I start learning pharmacology? You should keep in mind that when you enter a pharmaceutical lab you will be working closely with and under the supervision of a pharmaceutical rep. You will be able to learn by doing, so try to choose projects that allow you to learn in a hands-on manner. Your education will be better when you are allowed to participate in projects rather than learn by reading.

How do I start learning pharmacology?
The best way to get into a pharmaceutical lab is to get into an entry level position. These positions are typically in hospitals, nursing homes, research facilities, and pharmaceutical companies. You can get into one of these positions without completing a four-year degree. The higher level of education you earn, the more money you will make, and the more opportunities you will have.

# How can I memorize pharmacology drugs?

If you have ever tried to take an online pharma textbook or a loaded lecture from one of those on c Physiology then you will know that they are notoriously difficult to cram. This is because while they are informative and often times entertaining, the terms, names, and details used in them tend to blur together when trying to memorize them. There is a solution and it lies in the power of spaced repetition. Whether you use a drug name with the person who gave you the prescription, or you memorize it with the help of a graphing formula that can be found online, there are ways of making sure you remember each term and get through the entire pharmacology textbook in one sitting.

The first step to solving your pharmology homework is to determine if you will be taking a course in pharmacology at your local state university.
This step is very important, as many times students will take a course in their high school or college for the credit towards earning a pharma license.
If you will be taking this course at your local state university, they will more than likely require that you take a pre-licensing drug test before being allowed to enroll in the course.
In the pre-licensing test, the pharmacist will look over your academic history, your GPA's, and other factors to make sure that you are indeed ready for this challenging course. It is important to understand that even though you have passed the pre-licensing exam, you will still need to successfully complete the semester-long internship.

If you do not have a semester to work towards your degree, then the best way to study pharmacology in the comfort of your home is by using online resources. Although there are some significant advantages to studying online versus studying at a traditional university, there are also some major disadvantages. One of the major disadvantages is that there is not a group of peers that you will be able to study with. While you can study with other students who are in your same room, it will not be the same as having a large group of students around you.

Another way to study pharmacology is through the use of flashcards. Flashcards are a great way to memorize things quickly and effectively. The key to studying effectively with flashcards is to create lists of terms and key words, and then create pictures that represent these terms and key words on the card. For example, if you are going to study pharmacology class, you would want to have two pictures on each card that represent the chemical components found in these different compounds.

There are also several types of flashcards that you can buy specifically to help you study pharmacology.
These types of flashcards will often come with an illustration, or some sort of picture that represents the concept being taught.
One of the main advantages to these types of flashcards is that they are much more memorable than simply flipping through a dictionary or an index card. If you are taking a test when taking up the pharmacology course, having something to study under, such as these highly effective flashcards, will make the entire test take longer, and harder, due to the retention of the concepts.

A third method that you can use when learning to memorize the concepts of pharmacology is to draw them out using high yield jumbo pictures and pasted them on scrap paper, which is available from the local library. High yield jumbo pictures are pictures that are extremely large, and usually printed in color. These are easy to see and will easily keep the student's attention, as it is usually in bold lettering that will catch the student's eye and force them to read the phrase or word that is written on the card.

The last method that you can use to remember the information of pharmacology is through the use of anki (the cards with pictures on). An anki card is essentially just a square card, however, if you place a picture on the front and write the definition on the back, this is considered a personalized card. In recent years, many pharmacists have developed computer programs that can actually give you a personalized anki for your use. This makes it even easier to memorize, because the card is already tailored to the needs of the individual in question.

So, now you are probably wondering, "How can I memorize pharmacology drugs?" These are the questions you should ask yourself when asking yourself. Whether you use one of the three methods outlined above, or you find an effective memorization tool that you can keep in your pocket or briefcase at all times, the answer is simply to learn the material. This is probably the best way that you can be prepared for the licensing examination in your state.

# What are pharmacological concepts?

What are pharmacological concepts? These are the notions that underpin the way we treat medicine and, to a certain extent, how we think of it. A concept can be very complex and many of the modern approaches to treating diseases and improving health include these ideas. The field of medicine is deeply divided between those who believe that disease results from a defect in the human body and those who believe that disease is caused by a deficiency in the environment (natural environment). Neither side has a clear advantage when it comes to explaining the world around us.

Most people are familiar with concepts such as cause and effect, both of which are fundamental to our understanding of the medical world. Concepts such as cause and effect are not only used in medicine but also in physics, astronomy and chemistry. In many ways it is easier to grasp concepts like these than it is to grasp concepts such as metabolism or genetics. Indeed, many concepts in modern science are traceable to models based on models of the natural world.

What are the physiological effects of food? How are nutrients absorbed, metabolized and excreted? How do different bodies process information and how are different effects produced? This broad concept can be understood in very basic terms by understanding the effects of light on the retina and by studying the physiological functions of the nervous system.

What are the biochemical effects of drugs? When a drug is taken, it enters into the bloodstream where it works its way through the different cells and organs to reach the target area. It may stimulate one cell and inhibit the activity of another, altering the functionality of the target organ. We understand that the different levels of the brain must be balanced in order for a drug to have any effect.

What are the psychotherapeutic effects of drugs? They involve both physical and mental processes. The physical effects are often hard to measure because they are subtle. Therefore, the term psychosocial, which encompasses both physical and mental effects, is used to describe these effects of drugs on behavior.

What are the environmental pharmacological concepts? This includes both the physiological and the social aspects of drugs. For example, an abused substance is one that has been abused. This definition excludes illegal drugs such as cocaine, methamphetamine and ecstasy, but it includes prescription drugs that are misused by individuals for non-medical purposes. Examples include antidepressants, tranquilizers and painkillers. These concepts can also be used to explain social phenomena such as drug abuse among teenagers and among the young at college.

What are the pharmaceutical concepts? These are just a few of the many that exist when people start thinking about the various ways that drugs affect the body. They include dosage, action, mechanism, cause and effect, and toxicity. Dosage refers to how much of an agent is needed to produce the desired effect. Action describes how the drug gets to the target site and mechanism describes how the drug works once at the target site.

How do you learn these concepts? Generally, people learn about these concepts in two ways. They can learn them from textbooks or from other experts. However, some knowledge can be gained just by reading this article and becoming familiar with the major concepts.

The first concept explained above is the effect of a drug on the target site. An example of this would be the effect of caffeine on the central nervous system. The caffeine will affect the brain chemicals that control arousal and alertness to where they will remain when the person sleeps. This is just one example, but the result is the same.

The second concept is the mechanism of action. With a clear understanding of this concept, you will know how certain actions affect the target site and how those actions cause an effect in the rest of the body as well. You will know when and how to use certain medications with different effects depending on how they interact with other factors. For example, most people know that caffeine is a diuretic that increases urine output. What they don't know is how the diuretic is able to do this when it's used along with another substance or when it's consumed in combination with another medication.

Understanding what are pharmacological concepts? This is really quite simple. When you know how and why a substance works, you can then use that knowledge to help treat a disease. The next time someone asks you, "what are pharmaceutical concepts?" you'll be able to answer with confidence, " Concepts!"

Why is pharmacology so hard?

One of the most common questions that I get asked by my patients is "Why is pharmacology so hard?" I always tell them that there are many levels and detailed information about how these drugs work. Also, I have always been able to answer their questions with a lot of common sense and with a bit of patient education thrown in. However, some people still have trouble answering the question from a scientific point of view.

One of the reasons why is pharmacology is so difficult is because it requires you to learn so many details. The best way to do this is to take courses that are focused on pharmacology. The top 10 degree courses that focus on pharmacology are PharmD, MSN, BSN, and EdD. The first two are not mandatory, but if you want to get a job as a pharmacist you need to at least have a BSN or an EdD. I recommend that you choose the EdD first, because it will teach you all the important skills that you will use in your career. There are a lot of advantages to having an EdD including advancing your career and becoming more knowledgeable about the pharmaceutical industry.

The other reason why is pharmacology so hard is because it requires you to memorize a bunch of scientific terms that are used in the practice of pharmacy. One of the worst ways to learn this is by taking one of the many college level prepharmacy courses that are available. Even though prepharmacy courses cost money, they really don't give you enough information to pass the exam required for entry into a prepharmacy facility. So the only solution that is left to my students who would like to learn how to take prepharmacy exams is to get an EdD in pharmaceutical sciences. What makes this education program so great is that it will provide you with all the information that you need to pass your clinical experience exam. In my opinion, any educational program worth its salt will give you everything that you need to know to pass the clinical experience examination.

Another question that comes to mind when asking, "Why is pharmacology so hard?" is that pharmacology is the study of how different chemicals and compounds affect the human body and how these actions affect us from a physiological, psychological and behavioral level. These studies have been going on for decades and billions of dollars have been spent trying to understand them. This is not a difficult task by any stretch of the imagination, but it does take a huge amount of time and effort studying for the exams.

The first step in answering the question, "Why is pharmacology so hard?" is to try to memorize as much as you can. You should spend at least 4 hours each day studying pharmacology for nursing. It is very tempting to skip meals and avoid studying but that is the worst thing you can do for yourself because your body will get used to not feeling hungry and will inevitably work harder just to feel that food. In addition, you should avoid taking sleeping aids and other medications that will affect your ability to study effectively.

Next, you must know the concepts of pharmacology and anatomy. There are numerous levels of these concepts so you should find an English class that uses the terms fluently or find a teacher that has knowledge in these areas. There are two parts to the process of understanding pharmacology including Pharmacokinetics and Pharmacodynamics. Pharmacokinetics refers to how drugs are absorbed into the body and into the cells. Pharmacodynamics deals with the interactions of chemicals in the body and how these interact with one another to affect how the drug functions in the body.

Many individuals entering the field of pharmacology have a limited knowledge of the field because they did not start out as an undergraduate student majoring in chemistry, biology or other science major.
For those pharmacists who are choosing to major in clinical pharmacology, they must pass an exam that tests their knowledge of the physiology, anatomy and chemistry of human and animal tissues. Although pharmacognosy is becoming a more popular degree for many pharmacists, the exam process for this class is rigorous and those students who choose to major in this area must

take the examination very seriously. Only those students who have taken the previous areas of study and shown a significant level of competence in completing written applications and case studies will be considered for this class.

Finally, you must have extremely strong written and verbal communication skills. In order to apply pharmacognosy to a clinical practice setting, you need to be able to describe the properties of drugs, the physiological actions of them and how these actions affect the patient. As a result, you must know how to develop accurate written reports and narrative explanations of your findings. Furthermore, in the clinical setting, your patients must be able to understand the pharmacognosy behind your findings and why you reached the conclusion that a particular drug is effective in treating them. You cannot apply pharmacognosy to drug discovery if your patients do not understand what it means. It is important that the final output of your studies be well written, properly referenced and understood by your patients.

# What are pharmacological properties?

To answer this question a quick definition of Pharmacology is "the study of the chemistry, Physiology, and Biochemistry of drugs". In simpler terms it is the study of how drugs work on the human body. A pharmaceutical scientist is a person who is responsible for the development of new pharmaceuticals and analyzing their efficacy and safety. It is also his or her job to help develop standards of quality in the manufacturing and use of medical supplies. The scope of this article is to give you a basic understanding about what are pharmacological properties of a drug. This information will be valuable in making your decision when purchasing or considering treatments for any type of health condition.

Most people do not know that pharmaceutical companies make money by selling a lot of products that can help cure diseases. But they are also involved in discovering new pharmaceuticals that will help treat diseases that have not been discovered yet. The basic information about pharmacology that most people do not know is that it includes the study of how drugs interact with living systems such as the cells, tissues, organs, and blood flow. It also involves the study of how these systems are affected by exposure to health-related issues such as toxins, drugs, and chemicals.

The major function of pharmacology is the management of diseases. As such, pharmaceutical scientists are involved in finding out how a drug affects cells and how those changes affect the functioning of other organs. One example of such research scientist is the cytotoxic ologist. These cytotoxic ologists are responsible for determining the effects of drugs on cells and the effects that arise when cells are exposed to environmental hazards. Another area that falls under the purview of pharmacology is endocrinology.

All of the information that was mentioned above falls under the areas of pharmacology. These are all branches of pharmaceutical science. If you want to become a successful pharmaceutical researcher, you must be committed to complete a four year bachelor's degree, master's degree, or PhD in an area of interest to you.

As with many areas of study in the medical field, pharmaceutical research is divided into two major categories. These categories include biologically based drugs, known as biotechnological drugs, and pharmacologically based drugs, called pharmacotherapeutic agents. Both of these categories require rigorous and continuous research and development, as only through the advancements in technology can new medications be created. Pharmaceutical researchers look for a solution to a problem, rather than a simple cure. In other words, pharmacologists make the world safe for us by developing drugs that will cure the disease, rather than just treat the symptoms.

The world of pharmaceuticals has a few different faces, at the national, state, and regional levels. At the federal level, there are the Food and Drug Administration, or FDA, and the Drug Enforcement Administration, or DEA. These agencies regulate the manufacture and distribution of prescription and non-prescription drugs throughout the country. On a more localized level, there are the local zoning boards and health departments that administer the regulation of how pharmaceutical companies make money on their properties. The most important of all, however, are the pharmaceutical companies themselves which are responsible for developing the drugs and doing all the business with the appropriate authorities.

It is these companies that are the driving force behind what are 5 jobs of pharmacology. These jobs of pharmacology are also what make pharmology jobs so attractive to many pharmacists who are looking to get into the field of pharmaceutical research. Many pharmaceutical researchers begin their careers in the pharmaceutical industry by working in the area of research and development. Many of these pharmaceutical researchers and development officers spend much of their time doing research and development in the area of what are called metabolic systems, which are key to the synthesis and release of important compounds like polyphenols and flavonoids. In addition, a lot of time is spent trying to find new medications that will attack and even reverse the disease processes that lead to the onset of many health conditions.

On a more local level, pharmacologists also make an excellent living working in hospitals, nursing homes, clinics and doctor's offices as well as other health care facilities around the world. In fact, many pharmacists work in places like hospice, which provides care to those who have illness or who are terminally ill. There, they help patients who are suffering from various illnesses who cannot otherwise provide for themselves and their families. The job of a pharmacist, therefore, is to help improve the quality of life for those in need.

# Chapter 7

## What is autonomic pharmacology?

What is Autonomic Nervous System? It is a system which includes various nerves and organs that send signals throughout the body. Some of those nerves or organs are commonly known as'sympathetic','vagus' and 'urus'. These are branches of the sympathetic nervous system that cause pain, inflammation, and other symptoms. When these nerves are damaged, they can lead to a variety of health problems.

Why is it important to know what is autonomic? It's vital to understand this system since it affects how you feel on a day to day basis. If you are feeling good your nervous system will be working well. However, if you start to feel bad your nervous system will fail to work properly. This can have a variety of causes but one of the main reasons is due to the fact that the sympathetic nervous system will fail to properly regulate blood pressure and heart rate. In fact if this system isn't working correctly then it could cause a heart attack or stroke.

So now we know what is autonomic neuropathy? How is it caused? Well it's believed that when there is an imbalance in the brain's sensitivity to pain then an individual can suffer from a variety of health issues. Some of these include:

Headaches. This can happen if a person has a weak immune system. When the brain fails to send proper signals to the rest of the body then pain can be experienced. This could affect your teeth, tongue, limbs, and even the muscles in your face.

Lack of Pain. Another issue can occur if the nerves in the body don't receive proper signals from the brain. This can result in lack of pain, numbness, tingling, and other sensations.

If you have any of these symptoms then you may have what is called autonomic neuropathy. To find out if you do not have this condition the physician may perform a test called Bracheometry. This test can determine the location of where the dysfunction is located.

The test will measure the electrical resistance of the patient's body as they are stimulated by mild electric shocks. If there is an abnormality found the doctor will run a series of tests to find out what it is. Once the problem is found the physician can then make a treatment plan for the patient. This plan will involve the use of medication and possibly surgery to treat the issue. The medications used will depend on the severity of the condition of the patient.

The symptoms of what is autonomic neuropathy? If you feel like something is running in your body that you don't want to have, then you could be suffering with this problem. There are things that you can do to help prevent this from occurring, so don't fret. Being able to move your arm and your leg is a good way to keep this issue at bay.

What does it feel like when someone has this problem?
It can be described as tingling or numbing sensations in the legs or feet. Some people have a hard time walking after they get hurt. They also might be in excruciating pain. When a person experiences this they often become fearful and have a hard time relaxing. This can cause them to ignore pain in other parts of their body.

Why would someone develop this neuropathy anyway? There are many theories behind why this happens. Scientists have developed a few reasons why this occurs and they include things like genetics, heredity, and damage to nerve cells. Scientists aren't sure exactly why neuropathy happens but they have found that it is more common in some people than others.

If you need to know what is autonomic neuropathy? A patient may have peripheral neuropathy. In this case the doctor will do tests to find out if the patient's body is ready for the kind of treatment they need. If they find out the answer is yes, they can start treating the patient for neuropathy.

One common way to treat peripheral neuropathy is through acupuncture. In order to perform acupuncture, they will put the patient in a chair that has been electrically charged. Acupuncture works by removing the pain signals from the brain to allow the nerve to heal itself.

# What are the classes of autonomic drugs?

The definition of an Autonomic Nervous System (ANS) disorder is a condition where there is a disconnection or an inappropriate function of the nervous system. It is generally defined as an involuntary and continuous process by which the body restores itself to health when conditions warrant. There are three classes of drugs that fall within the category of Autonomic Nervous Drugs. They are; the beta blockers, anti-convulsant, and the opioids. Each class displays signs and symptoms which include; restlessness, irritability, chronic pain, lack of concentration, hyperactivity, and many more.

The use of Drugs A, B, C and D as treatment modalities has been shown to produce relief from the symptoms of many diseases including allergies, arthritis, asthma, chronic fatigue, insomnia, migraine headaches, nausea, vomiting, sexual dysfunction, urinary tract infections, vision problems, and much more. This class includes over two hundred medications. These drugs affect the functions of the digestive, respiratory, cardiovascular and genitor-urinary systems. The effects of these drugs can either be relaxing of disruptive. Some of the common classifications of Drugs are mentioned below.

Antidepressant drugs are the most commonly used drugs for treating Depression. These drugs act on the neurotransmitters of the brain which are responsible for controlling emotion. The effects are reported to be almost instant and some reports are of up to four weeks of relief. The relief is produced by increasing serotonin levels in the brain which in turn improves the feelings of well-being. It also helps reduce sleep disorders and tension which helps prevent depression.

Anti-anxiety drugs are also very popular and have similar effects to that of the antidepressant drugs. The main difference lies in the antiaquital properties of this drug that blocks or slows down panic and anxiety attacks. The slowing of the attack prevents the stimuli from reaching the brain which causes a relaxed feeling. This leads to better sleep and relaxation.

Opioids are the most widely prescribed drugs. They are effective in relieving the pain caused by irritable bowel syndrome, especially in children. The opioids have strong sedative effects which make it easier for the patients to get to sleep. Some of the classifications of drugs include opium, hydrocodone, hydromorphone, and oxycodone. Opiates are also the most used for chronic pain management in the United States.

Narcotic drugs produce long lasting but temporary effects of euphoria. The euphoric effects of this class of drug are often experienced during the early morning hours. Later the effects of the drug wear off causing sleepiness and drowsiness which make it difficult for an individual to fall asleep.

Sleep medications such as tranquilizers, anti-convulsant, and sedatives are used to treat conditions like insomnia, sleep apnea, and narcolepsy. These drugs help individuals fall asleep and stay asleep. Some of the classifications of drugs are benzodiazepines, azapirones, nonbenzodiazepine hypnotics, antidepressants, nonbenzodiazepine sedatives, and narcotics. They differ from each other in their effect on the central nervous system, actions on the circulatory system, and their ability to induce or reduce sleep.

Studies conducted on what are the classes of autonomic drugs? have shown that sleep apnea is associated with low levels of dopamine in the brain and low levels of melatonin in the body. Other studies conducted on what are the classes of autonomic drugs? have indicated that people who are suffering from obstructive sleep apnea are those who consume alcohol, smoke, and eat large meals before going to bed.

Dopamine, a neurotransmitter, plays an important role in the body's regulation of arousals, the number of times an individual spontaneously goes into a deep sleep state. Low levels of dopamine and melatonin lead to sleep disorders, including insomnia, sleep apnea, narcolepsy, and polyominos, which include occurrences when the person does not enter a deep sleep state. What are the classes of autonomic drugs? are a category of drugs that block the action of acetylcholine in the body. Acetylcholine is the neurotransmitter that is responsible for initiating the conscious movement of the muscles and coordinating eye movements during the night.

The last two classes of drugs are the non-benzodiazepine sedatives and narcotics. Naxal one and Zolpidem are nonbenzodiazepines that slow down or stop the body's reflexive response to anxiety or stress. They can thus reduce the occurrence of sleep apnea. However, they are not considered very effective in relieving the problem on their own since they do not affect consciousness. Benzodiazepines, however, work by altering the level of consciousness and thereby reducing or eliminating the effects of anxiety and stress. These drugs should only be used under the strict supervision of a medical practitioner.

So, what are the classes of autonomic drugs? sleep apnea is caused when a person's respiratory system does not regulate its own temperature. This can happen because of physical or psychological conditions. It can result in the abrupt awakening of an otherwise sound sleep partner.

# What are the 3 divisions of the autonomic nervous system?

The three major parts of the autonomic nervous system are the parasympathetic nervous system, the sympathetic nervous system, and the gastrointestinal (GI) nervous system. These three parts work together to keep the body's normal functions under control. In order for us to have a full life, these three parts of the nervous system need to be functioning correctly. If one or more of these organs is malfunctioning, we experience symptoms such as: fatigue, anxiety, irritability, and many other common conditions that disrupt our day to day living. This article will discuss the 3 divisions of the autonomic nervous system.

The Parasympathetic division of the autonomic nervous system controls the body's relaxation and the fight or flight response. This division is divided into two sub divisions called the sympathetic division which includes the adrenalin gland, and the noradrenalin glands. The sympathetic division of the body has a direct effect on cardiac function, and its activity is activated when the body detects danger. When this division is injured or corrupted, however, it can malfunction and result in cardiac arrest or death.

The Sympathetic division of the autonomic nervous system makes an effort to control breathing and heart rate through the respiratory system, and it also controls the involuntary nervous system (such as the immune system and the digestive system).
This division has a direct impact on cardiac output and its control, and is activated during times of stress. This division is divided into two sub divisions: the cardiac muscle (the muscle that controls the heart) and the sympathetic ganglion. The cardiac muscle is divided into two branches: the coronary muscle (which supplies the heart) and the coronary artery.

The Perceptively-Sensed (or Afferent) division of the autonomic nervous system controls what we see. This division is activated when our bodies think there is a threat or some kind of harm. This is why we often feel pain or stress when we are injured. For example, the feeling of pain is produced by the division at the endocardium, which receives sensory information from the blood vessels supplying the skin surface.

The Sympathetic division of the nervous system directly influences the cardiac output, which it subdivides into three types: Sympathetic Nervous System, sympathetic axon reflex, and other. The Sympathetic Nervous System produces the 'fight or flight' response, which is triggered when our bodies detect a threat. This is used by the sympathetic division to increase cardiac output when the situation requires it. The Sympathetic Axon Reflex commands the release of the hormones epinephrine and cortisol to the adrenal glands, which then secrete these hormones into the bloodstream to stimulate the heart to beat faster.

The Parasympathetic division of the nervous system controls the body's reaction to no stimuli. Parasympathetic Nervous System produces the 'relaxant' or relaxing response. The Parasympathetic Nervous System is activated by no physical stimuli such as exercise, stress, or even a cold. When a person is stressed, it releases the 'fight or flight' hormone into the bloodstream, which in turn stimulates the parasympathetic nervous system to secrete more adrenaline into the blood.

Last but not least is the Intrauterine System. The IUS runs between the brain and the internal organs. It connects the visceral (stomach) and parasympathetic (heart) nerves. It also connects the brainstem with the abdominal organs. This division of the nervous system controls important organs such as the gastrointestinal tract, the reproductive system, the blood pressure regulation, and the immune system.

These three divisions of the nervous system are crucial in keeping an individual healthy. However, one must understand that these functions are not independent of each other. Each division performs a specific function when needed and may rely on the other divisions for additional information. A person may have a perfectly functioning division one day, but may need the other division for some processes to be completed. Understanding what are the three divisions of the autonomic nervous system is essential to having optimal health.

# What are examples of autonomic responses?

What are examples of autonomic responses? When you think about it, there are many different types of responses that occur in the body. They all have a purpose and are necessary for the proper functioning of the body. For example, when your heart beats it is an autonomic response to a signal from the brain that something is going on in your body. This is one of the most common of all responses. An individual who is not in a deep sleep has their heart rate speeding up due to the fact they are alert to their surroundings.

When people are driving they may experience a different type of reaction. This could be due to a lack of relaxation or because of a mental block due to the road conditions. Some individuals have no problem relaxing while others are tensed up, anxious or in a panic mode.

All of these examples can occur without the individual knowing. However, the cause and effect are often the same. For instance, some people react to certain stimuli with a sense of anxiety or fear. These can actually be examples of fear responses.

The next example is shaking your head. Some individuals feel a sensation that they should not be. For example, if the person is shaking their head from excitement, it could be considered a positive response. However, if they are shaking their head from sadness or pain, it could be considered a negative response.

Another example is laughing. There are people who find it funny to laugh. This is actually a physiological response to a stimulus. However, some people find this to be a negative response. For instance, if the individual is laughing at a sad situation, they will be showing an example of depression.

A classic example is the fight or flight response. If you ever had to make a choice to fight or to flight during a flight, which would you choose? Chances are that you would choose the fight response. This could involve increased heart rate and blood pressure, sweating, fast breathing, numbness in the hands, and even confusion.

What are examples of autonomic responses? They exist in all of us. They are unconscious responses that we do automatically without thinking. They serve a purpose by letting us know that something is going on. Yet, sometimes they can get out of hand and lead to some pretty wild behavior.

For instance, in one study, male subjects who were asked to dig their own grave took longer to do so than those who were simply asked to empty the grave. The reason for this was because the person had to control their unconscious reaction. In most cases, the unconscious mind will take care of the situation until we have a chance to react appropriately. The examples listed above are just a few that you might encounter.

What are the other examples of autonomic reactions? One reaction that you may encounter is to jump or to jog when walking. Jogging is an example of an autonomic response, as well as falling down from a great height.

What causes these reactions? During the dive you experience a very strong and fast heart rate. As a result, you may be breathing so hard you can hear your lungs choking. The examples listed above all involve a sudden, forceful movement of your body. You cannot control every movement of your body at the same time.

How can this information be useful to you? This type of training is very useful to pilots and astronauts. If you are working in a manufacturing setting, for instance, you are required to follow very specific guidelines every day. By learning how the body reacts to specific scenarios, you can become more aware of problems and you can make adjustments before they happen.

If you are interested in studying hypnosis and how it applies to your everyday life, the information above will be invaluable. It will take some time and effort to understand, but you will find that you become calmer and more centered by learning how the body responds to certain situations. An important part of this training is self-hypnosis. If you cannot afford professional classes, there are a number of resources available to you on the internet. What are examples of autonomic reactions?

# Chapter 8

## Psychiatric Pharmacology

Psychiatric pharmacology deals with the action of medications within the body in controlling the serotonin system. Serotonin is considered one of the major neurotransmitters in the brain that controls mood, appetite, sleep, sexual function and other body functions. As a result of its vital role in the body, when there is an imbalance involving the levels of this neurotransmitter, the result is psychiatric disorder or illness. In most cases, people who suffer from psychiatric disorder or schizophrenia often show abnormal activity within the brain.

This disorder usually includes hallucinations, paranoia, compulsions, depression and mania. Psychotic episodes may also occur along with these symptoms. While using medications for treating these symptoms, patients are directed to use only those medications that contain ingredients that are aimed at controlling the chemical interaction between certain antidepressants and serotonin in the brain.

For patients with psychiatric disorder, doctors will often prescribed various types of antidepressant medications including serotonin reuptake inhibitors (SSRIs), tricyclics and monoamine oxidase inhibitors (MAOIs).
These medications are able to successfully reduce symptoms and help control the body's chemical reactions to stress and other events that can trigger the symptoms of this disorder. But sometimes, these medications are not able to do this task and some antidepressants have been known to cause further problems for the patient. This is why it is very important for doctors to monitor their patients closely and find out which medications are causing more problems and if there are any drugs present that should be avoided.

Another important area of psychiatric pharmacology is the use of anticonvulsants. These drugs are widely used to treat epileptic seizures, which is associated with abnormal behavior in the patient such as convulsions and loss of consciousness. However, these medications can also have some serious side effects. If the dosage is improperly determined, it can also result to a more severe reaction than what is originally expected. In fact, these type of drugs have been known to cause coma and even death in extremely severe cases.

Many people also choose to use medications called antidepressants or selective serotonin reuptake inhibitors (SSRIs) to treat their psychiatric conditions. While these medications can have good effects on the patient, they also have very negative effects especially when the dose is not properly administered. Individuals who take these medications must be carefully monitored by their doctors so that there will be no overdose of the medication or when the right amount is not taken at all. Some antidepressants can also be very addictive and can result to other harmful behaviors if they are abused.

Another type of medication commonly used to treat psychiatric illnesses is tranquilizers or sedatives.
These are usually prescribed to relieve severe anxiety, depression or panic attacks. However, these medications can also have very negative effects and can cause cardiac arrest or even death. It is therefore imperative that medical professionals know how to correctly administer these medications and that an emergency doctor should also be immediately seen in case of an emergency.

Finally, another common type of psychiatric medication is antidepressants or monoamine oxidase inhibitors (MAOIs). These medications can either have specific effects on one chemical in the brain or they can target many different chemical within the brain at once. For example, Zoloft, an antidepressant is known to work on serotonin functions by increasing the amount of the hormone norepinephrine while Prozac works on dopamine functions. MAOIs have been known to increase the brain chemical norepinephrine which has proven to be useful for people with obsessive compulsive disorders.

As you can see, there are many different medications used in psychiatric pharmacology. However, all medications should be properly approved for treatment before they can be used. There are a lot of side effects associated with these medications which includes drowsiness, nausea, and sleepiness. It is therefore important that patients who suffer from psychiatric conditions be aware of the side effects that can come along with a particular medication and be sure to consult their physicians before they begin a course of medication. Although medication can provide some relief from symptoms of psychiatric conditions, it is not appropriate for everyone and patients need to be monitored closely by their doctors to make sure the medications do not cause more harm than good.

# What are the 7 classifications of psychotropic medications?

Psychotropic medications refer to any drug that can affect your brain and the way it works. These are used to treat mental illnesses such as depression, schizophrenia, bipolar disorder, post traumatic stress disorder, and even attention deficit disorder in children. So how do these drugs work? Medications in this category affect brain chemistry to alter it. They alter the transmission of nerve cell information to and from the brain. These changes result in a change in the person's mood, thought patterns, and behaviors.

A few categories fall under the heading of psychotropic medications classified as "stimulants". These include Ritalin, Adderall, and Cylert. These medicines cause similar effects as the original stimulant, which is amphetamine. The main difference is that they don't stay in the brain long enough to have their full effect.

Another classification of psychotropic medications is referred to as "cholinergic". Medications in this category include benzodiazepines, tranquilizers, and antidepressants. It is important to note that there is considerable debate surrounding the link between cholinergic antidepressants and retardation of brain development in children. Many in the medical community believe there are serious side effects with these types of treatment, and are not recommended for children under the age of 12.

One classification of psychotropic drug is referred to as a "mood stabilizer". This includes drugs such as Brahmi (Bacopa monnieri), Shankhpushpi (Convolvulus pluricaulis), Vacha (Acorus calamus), Jatamansi (Nardostachys jatamansi), Ashwagandha (Withania somnifera), Shatavari (Asparagus racemosus), Kushmand (Benincasa hispida), Pippali (Piper longum) and Kushmand (Benincasa hispida). It is believed that these drugs can effectively treat anxiety and depression in children and adolescents. However, it should be noted that there is a great deal of controversy surrounding the effects of these medications.

The last classification, called an "anti-psychotic" is believed by many to be the most effective when treating children with mental health issues. Anti psychotic medications are usually given to children who have committed acts of violence or self harm. However, there is some controversy surrounding this classification. Some researchers feel that children, particularly those who are diagnosed with schizophrenia, are unable to process anxiety and stress properly, so they inappropriately respond to them. However, many children benefit from this type of psychotropic treatment. Other children are able to use this treatment to reduce symptoms of anxiety and depression and remain relatively calm overall.

This last classification, known as an "anti-anxiety" psychotropic drug, is given to children who are suffering from severe symptoms of anxiety and panic attacks. The main goal of this classification is to prevent the development of phobias or the occurrence of panic attacks. Commonly prescribed anti-anxiety medications include benzodiazepines and azapirones. These types of medications are not used to treat obsessive-compulsive disorders, such as autism, dementia, and schizophrenia.

If you or someone you love has been diagnosed with a mental health problem or illness, it is very important that you discuss your concerns with your medical doctor. This discussion will likely lead to a referral to a psychologist or psychiatrist. There are three main types of psychotropic medications available for children and adolescents. These include tricyclic antidepressants (TCA), monoamine oxidase inhibitors (MAOIs) and selective serotonin reuptake inhibitors (SSRIs). Children can be prescribed one or more of these drugs depending on the severity of their symptoms. While some children receive all of these treatments, others only receive one or two of these treatments.

The classification of psychotropic medications is designed to help provide relief and treatment for those who suffer from a mental illness. Some of the most common psychotropic drugs recommended for children include Risperdal (Risperdal), Anafranil (Clomipramine), Furosemide (Prozac), Oxcarbazepine (Sertraline), Clozapine (Clozapine), fluoxetine (Prozac), and Selective Serotonin Reuptake Inhibitors (SSRIs). It is important that you discuss your child's case with a qualified medical professional, such as a child psychologist, before starting any psychotropic drug treatment. Your child's needs will be the number one factor in determining which drug regimen will be best for your child.

# What is a psychiatric pharmacologist?

A psychiatric pharmacist, or psychiatrist, is a medical doctor who provides psychiatric treatment to patients. The most common medications that a psychiatrist will prescribe include anti-psychotics such as olanzapine and clozapine; antidepressants like sertraline and venapro; anxiolytics like perphenazine and tricyclics; and antipsychotic drugs, including Risperdal and olanzapine. Some psychiatrists work with a team to treat their patients, while others will work entirely on their own. There are also other physicians who work in close conjunction with a psychiatrist. In this article, we'll look at what a psychiatric pharmacist does, and some of the key things they should be certified in.

Generally speaking, a psychiatrist is licensed by the state in which they practice, and will receive a Master's degree in Psychology, Medical Science, or Pharmaceutical Administration. After obtaining their doctorate degree, they will generally take additional years of education, training, and study in order to qualify as a practicing psychiatrist in the state of their choice. In many states, they will also be required to pass the Certified Psychiatric Ser counselor examination. Once they have met all of these requirements, they will be board certified. This certification process differs from state to state, but in general, once you meet the criteria to sit for the exam, you must practice for two years in order to gain your license.

A psychiatrist works closely with their physician in order to formulate the most effective medications possible. They are responsible for ensuring that an appropriate mix of dosages is found, and that the correct dosage is prescribed. This means that each patient's medications used is unique, and requires the appropriate amount. Not only that, but the medications used will vary depending on the severity of the condition that a patient is diagnosed with. A psychiatrist's job can be extremely stressful, and can involve working closely with patients who suffer from serious mental disorders.

When considering what is a psychiatric pharmacist?, the most common question that is asked is regarding psychotropic medications. These are the medications used to treat most mental disorders, including schizophrenia and bipolar disorder. Depending on the severity of the condition that a patient is diagnosed with, these medication sessions can range from one to several times a day, and can last up to six months. Some of the most common psychotropic medications used by pharmacists include antipsychotic drugs, antidepressants, and mood stabilizers.

Another question that is frequently asked is regarding non-psychiatric, or over the counter, medications that may be prescribed by a psychiatrist. These may include things like cold and flu treatments, as well as pain management medications. While it is rare, some pharmacists may also prescribe medications used for contraception purposes. There are many reasons why a person may be referred to a psychiatrist, including an overdose of certain types of medications, chemical imbalances related to depression or other mental conditions, or the need to treat a physical problem such as a physical defect.

Other questions that are commonly asked about what is a psychiatric pharmacist?
One of the most important factors to understand is that most states require that pharmacists have completed a specific number of hours of continuing education in order to maintain their license.
This education can take many forms, but is almost always required for licensure in any state in the United States. While some states may also require that they have taken courses on the use of psychiatric drugs, it is not required that they have actually received any specific training on these drugs. These questions and answers relating to what is a psychiatric pharmacist can be found by looking at the specific requirements of the specific state where the pharmacist works.

There are many benefits to working as a psychiatric pharmacist. In addition to the fact that you will have a lot of different jobs that you are involved in during your career, you will also find that you are working in an environment that has a good reputation for treating mental illnesses and diseases. If you work in a doctor's office, hospital or other health care facility, you will know that you are in the position to be surrounded by highly educated people who have been trained to provide treatment for various mental disorders. You may also work with people who are considered to be addicted to medications or alcohol. If you work in a pharmacy or another place where there are powerful medications being used to treat these ailments, you will be working with people who are addicted to these medications, as well as to alcohol.

As you can see, the answer to the question, what is a psychiatric pharmacist? can change based upon the type of facility in which you work. Regardless of the type of environment you work in, you will be involved in health care and pharmaceuticals information regarding medications and mental illnesses.

# What are the drugs used in psychiatry?

If you or a loved one has been diagnosed with an addiction to alcohol or drugs, it is imperative that you know what are the drugs used in psychiatry? Detoxification, the process of clearing a person's body of chemicals and substances that are abusing it, is a necessary step for every addict. This is also a necessary first step towards recovery. However, one should never forget that rehab is not just a quick fix, but a permanent change to a person's life that will require years of support and supervision.

Amongst the drugs used in psychiatry, those dealing with anxiety disorders are particularly vulnerable to being adversely affected by the effects of these medications. Various antidepressants have been developed to treat this condition, which includes selective serotonin reuptake inhibitors (SSRIs), atypical antipsychotics and tricyclics. The problem with these medications is that they tend to have a numbing effect, which can prevent the person affected from responding to therapy. However, the use of SSRIs and TCA is particularly useful in combating the withdrawal symptoms experienced when an alcoholic or drug addict tries to quit.

While TCA and SSRIs are relatively slow to produce effects, they are highly effective when it comes to controlling urges to relapse. The use of benzodiazepines, however, should be considered cautiously, as this group of drugs can cause a build-up of tolerance, which means that the user would have to consume more drugs to achieve the same effect. Some of the benzodiazepines most often used are alprazolam, haloperidol, lorazepam, fluphenazine and temazepam. These drugs should only be administered under close medical supervision to minimize the risk of dependency.

Antipsychotic drugs are another group of drugs that are frequently used in psychiatry. They are often prescribed in cases where a person is experiencing symptoms of mania, which can result in hallucinations and delusions. This group of drugs includes Risperdal, olanzapine, quetiapine, clomipramine and otroctol. antipsychotic medicines are most effective when used in conjunction with other forms of treatment, such as behavioral therapy. Because of this, care must be taken so that the patient receives sufficient amount of medical care while under the influence of these medications.

Antipsychotic medicines are usually used to treat conditions that affect moods, including depression, psychosis, mania, bi-polar disorder, obsessive-compulsive disorders and schizophrenia. They also play an important role in reducing symptoms of anxiety and panic disorders. When a patient uses antipsychotic drugs to treat his or her anxiety disorders, it is known as benzodiazepine use. What are the drugs used in psychiatry used in the treatment of anxiety disorders?

Selective Serotonin Reuptake Inhibitors (SSRIs) are a class of medications that help treat obsessive-compulsive disorders. This category includes such widely used medications as Paxil, Prozac, Zoloft and Celexa. What are the drugs used in psychiatry used in the treatment of obsessive-compulsive disorders? SSRIs are one type of drug that works by preventing serotonin from being reabsorbed into the brain. They are used in combination with neuroleptic drugs in cases where the patient's ability to take medication is impaired due to other medical causes.

Nefazodone, or Norpramin, is a generic name for non-benzodiazepine sedatives.
It is commonly used in the treatment of Parkinson's disease and is part of the triptan family of drugs used in psychiatry. What are the drugs used in psychiatry used in the treatment of depression? Monoamine oxidase inhibitors (MAOIs) work to reduce the number of reactive chemicals in the brain that cause depression.

What are the drugs used in psychiatry used in the treatment of anxiety? General tranquilizers such as Klonopin, Valium, Ativan and Xanax are often used in the treatment of panic attacks and anxiety disorders. What are the drugs used in psychiatry used in the treatment of bipolar disorder? Affective-tics are a category of anti-depressants and benzodiazepines used in the treatment of mania. What are the drugs used in psychiatry used in the treatment of schizophrenia?

# Best Pharmacology

With the hope to assist you in your career aspirations, have compiled the best pharmacology flash cards for nursing students. Nursing as a career is one of the most attractive professions in today's world. Due to its nature as a medical profession, many people prefer it over other careers due to its high pay scale, job security, and benefits like paternity leave and pension plans. Pharmacy, on the other hand, is a highly competitive career that requires energetic, intelligent people who have sharp skills and are able to develop innovative solutions to patients' problems.

However, there is one thing that makes pharmacy more challenging than nursing pharmacology: the limited availability of medical knowledge and experience that comes with a degree in Pharmacy.

As a result, most aspiring pharmacists have to rely on a host of textbooks to keep up to date with new concepts and medication-related developments. Even if they have access to relevant information, they are usually unable to incorporate it into their clinical practice as a nurse. For those students who are already in the field but aspire to apply for a position of nursing, this could be an avenue that they could explore.

The best way for a student to make sure that they will have enough and relevant pharmacology textbooks under their belt is to acquire one or two textbooks related to the pharmaceutical field. These books are typically helpful in supplementing a student's knowledge as they delve deeper into the intricacies of pharmaceuticals and its application in their clinical practice. They offer basic understanding of drugs in terms of how they work and what their various properties are. They also teach students the basic principles of pharmacology, anatomy and physiology, and basic functions of body systems. All of these fundamentals are crucial in properly studying the drugs and their effects on the body.

One of the best pharmacology books that you can acquire is From Idea to Discovery by Russell Stutely. This book tackles important issues in the world of medication and pharmaceuticals. Some of the topics covered include drug design, development of drugs, introduction of new drugs, regulatory issues and medical ethics. It addresses how changes in medication lead to adverse reactions and what to do as a health care professional when such changes occur. The book also tackles important legal issues that arise when taking a particular medication.

Another highly recommended book on pharmacology is The Art of Success by Jack Canfield. The Art of Success is written in an extremely easy to understand language. The book contains information on how you can choose the right type of drugs for your patients, the most effective types, and how to ensure that they are taken correctly. Additionally, the book contains interesting case studies and illustrations which show just how simple changes in the way that you administer medication can lead to dramatically improved results.

For those students studying pharmacology at colleges or universities, there are many textbooks available to aid in the process. The Best Pharmacology Flashcards and study guides from Dr. Nicholas Kastan, J.D are both extremely easy to use and are among the best books for students who want to learn about pharmacology in a quick and easy format. The Best Pharmacology Flashcards contains information on the various types of flashcards that students should use while studying. The flash cards feature information on over seventy different diseases and ailments, along with explanations of how to interpret the data provided on the flashcards.

The Best Pharmacology Study Guide is another very popular version of the flashcard series. Like the flashcard edition, the study guide includes information on how to read the labels of medications, as well as the scientific names of the different ingredients within the medication. The study guide also includes information on how to determine the dosage of each ingredient, how to combine ingredients, and key details regarding each medication type. The study guide also provides students with detailed examples on how to complete basic pharmacology tasks, as well as how to create a pharmacist prescription.

For students who are interested in learning about a particular area of pharmacology, the Best Pharmacology Flashcards and study guides offer a great way to learn the material. Rather than being in a classroom, these types of flashcards and study pharmacology guides allow students to access helpful content whenever they want or need it. For students who are taking online classes, the Best Pharmacology Flashcards and study pharmacology guides are invaluable tools. For students who can't afford the materials that would normally be needed to take an online class, the Best Pharmacology Flashcards and study pharmacology guides provide an affordable alternative to traditional courses.

www.ingramcontent.com/pod-product-compliance
Lightning Source LLC
Chambersburg PA
CBHW081825200326
41597CB00023B/4390